How to access the supplemental web resource

We are pleased to provide access to a web resource that supplements your textbook, *Athletic Taping, Bracing, and Casting, Fourth Edition.* This resource offers checklists that detail the main steps an athletic training student must demonstrate to show competency in 56 casting, splinting, and taping procedures and 47 video clips that help to illustrate the techniques presented in the text.

Accessing the web resource is easy!
Follow these steps if you purchased a new book:

1. Visit **www.HumanKinetics.com/AthleticTapingBracingAndCasting**.

2. Click the <u>fourth edition</u> link next to the corresponding fourth edition book cover.

3. Click the Sign In link on the left or top of the page. If you do not have an account with Human Kinetics, you will be prompted to create one.

4. If the online product you purchased does not appear in the Ancillary Items box on the left of the page, click the Enter Key Code option in that box. Enter the key code that is printed at the right, including all hyphens. Click the Submit button to unlock your online product.

5. After you have entered your key code the first time, you will never have to enter it again to access this product. Once unlocked, a link to your product will permanently appear in the menu on the left. For future visits, all you need to do is sign in to the textbook's website and follow the link that appears in the left menu!

→ Click the Need Help? button on the textbook's website if you need assistance along the way.

How to access the web resource if you purchased a used book:

You may purchase access to the web resource by visiting the text's website, **www.HumanKinetics.com/AthleticTapingBracingAndCasting**, or by calling the following:

800-747-4457 . . . . U.S. customers
800-465-7301 . . . . .Canadian customers
+44 (0) 113 255 5665 . . . . European customers
217-351-5076 . . . . .International customers

For technical support, send an email to:
support@hkusa.com . . . . U.S. and international customers
info@hkcanada.com . . . . Canadian customers
academic@hkeurope.com . . . . European customers

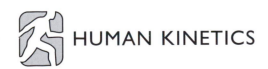
HUMAN KINETICS

05-2018

Product: Athletic Taping, Bracing, and Casting, Fourth Edition, web resource

Key code: PERRIN-AUJIGW-OSG

This unique code allows you access to the web resource.

Access is provided if you have purchased a new book. Once submitted, the code may not be entered for any other user.

HUMAN KINETICS WEB RESOURCE

Athletic Taping, Bracing, and Casting

FOURTH EDITION

David H. Perrin, PhD, FNATA

University of Utah

Ian A. McLeod, PA-C, ATC

Northern Arizona University

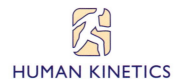

HUMAN KINETICS

Library of Congress Cataloging-in-Publication Data

Names: Perrin, David H., 1954- author. | McLeod, Ian A., 1975- author.
Title: Athletic taping, bracing, and casting / David H. Perrin, PhD,
  FNATA, University of Utah, Ian A. McLeod, MEd, MS, PA-C, ATC, Northern Arizona
  University.
Other titles: Athletic taping and bracing
Description: Fourth edition. | Champaign, IL : Human Kinetics, [2019] |
  Revised edition of: Athletic taping and bracing / David H. Perrin. 3rd ed.
  2012. | Includes bibliographical references.
Identifiers: LCCN 2017055720 (print) | LCCN 2017056398 (ebook) | ISBN
  9781492567677 (enhanced ebook) | ISBN 9781492554905 (print)
Subjects: LCSH: Sports injuries--Treatment. | Bandages and bandaging.
Classification: LCC RD97 (ebook) | LCC RD97 .P47 2019 (print) | DDC
  617.1/027--dc23
LC record available at https://lccn.loc.gov/2017055720

ISBN: 978-1-4925-5490-5 (print)

This book is a revised edition of *Athletic Taping and Bracing, Third Edition,* published in 2012 by Human Kinetics, Inc.

The web addresses cited in this text were current as of March 2018, unless otherwise noted.

Senior Acquisitions Editor: Joshua J. Stone; **Developmental and Managing Editor:** Carly S. O'Connor; **Copyeditor:** Pamela S. Johnson; **Permissions Manager:** Dalene Reeder; **Graphic Designer:** Dawn Sills; **Cover Designer:** Keri Evans; **Cover Design Associate:** Susan Rothermel Allen; **Photograph (cover):** © Human Kinetics; **Photographs (interior):** © Human Kinetics, unless otherwise noted; **Photo Production Coordinator:** Amy M. Rose; **Photo Production Manager:** Jason Allen; **Senior Art Manager:** Kelly Hendren; **Illustrations:** © Human Kinetics, unless otherwise noted; **Printer:** Premier Print Group

We thank A.T. Still University in Mesa, AZ, for assistance in providing the location for the photo shoot for this book.

The video contents of this product are licensed for educational public performance for viewing by a traditional (live) audience, via closed circuit television, or via computerized local area networks within a single building or geographically unified campus. To request a license to broadcast these contents to a wider audience—for example, throughout a school district or state, or on a television station—please contact your sales representative (**www.HumanKinetics.com/SalesRepresentatives**).

Printed in the United States of America   10 9 8 7 6 5 4 3 2 1

Human Kinetics
P.O. Box 5076
Champaign, IL 61825-5076
Website: www.HumanKinetics.com

In the United States, email info@hkusa.com or call 800-747-4457.
In Canada, email info@hkcanada.com.
In the United Kingdom/Europe, email hk@hkeurope.com.

For information about Human Kinetics' coverage in other areas of the world,
please visit our website: **www.HumanKinetics.com**

E7098

Contents

Preface

Mastering the art and science of athletic taping, bracing, and casting requires athletic training students to develop the psychomotor skills associated with the craft and learn the scientific principles that guide their application. Educators seeking to convey this dual emphasis face the daunting task of teaching students the anatomical architecture of the major joints and muscle groups as well as specific taping, bracing, and casting techniques associated with particular injuries.

Athletic Taping, Bracing, and Casting, Fourth Edition, was written as both a guide for instructors and an aid to students. The book includes concise descriptions of anatomy and detailed anatomical illustrations (of the quality usually found in advanced anatomy texts) integrated with discussions of injury mechanisms and more than 550 photographs depicting the taping, bracing, and casting techniques for each major joint and body region. The taping, bracing, and casting techniques covered in this book include traditional taping as well as rigid strap taping, elastic kinesiology taping, and techniques for immobilization with casting and splinting. We believe that this approach will not only encourage skill development but also help ensure familiarity with the underlying anatomical landscapes.

This book focuses on the taping, bracing, casting, and splinting techniques athletic trainers are most likely to apply in clinical practice. Athletic training students can easily become overwhelmed by an excessive presentation of techniques they are unlikely to use in the field. The techniques presented in this book not only are those most frequently applied in clinical practice but also can be easily mastered during a one-semester laboratory.

Because exercise plays an equally important role in a patient's safe return to competition, we include a presentation of the basic stretching and strengthening exercises associated with specific injuries. Although these exercises should not replace other therapeutic methods, they can help the rehabilitated patient maintain strength and flexibility. The methods we present apply to the patient who has completed a rehabilitation program and met the criteria for returning to competition. Our approach to this material emphasizes that athletic taping, bracing, and casting and the associated exercises serve as an adjunct, rather than a panacea, to the patient's total rehabilitation. By using this multifaceted treatment approach we can minimize a patient's chance of reinjury. Be advised, however, that rehabilitation and therapeutic exercise are disciplines distinct from the treatments that we discuss in this book.

ORGANIZATION

Chapter 1 establishes athletic taping, bracing, casting, and splinting within the context of the multifaceted practice of athletic training. The chapter stresses the importance of learning anatomy as the foundation to athletic taping and understanding the effect of taping on athletic performance. To set the stage for the techniques presented in this book, the concept and importance of evidence-based practice as an integral part of the decision-making process when interacting with patients is introduced. Students will also learn the necessity of following the rules of the governing sport organizations for the application of tape, braces, and casts. Rigid strapping tape and elastic kinesiology tape are also introduced as alternatives to traditional tape. The precautions and application guidelines for these alternatives set the stage for the techniques to be illustrated in subsequent chapters. The concepts underlying the application of casts and splints are also introduced.

Chapters 2 through 7 address and illustrate anatomy and injury mechanisms; traditional, rigid strap, and elastic kinesiology taping and bracing techniques; and associated stretching and strengthening exercises for each region of the body. Where appropriate, common fractures and techniques for applying casts and splints for immobilization are also included. Chapter 2 focuses on the foot-ankle-leg complex and, besides presenting several techniques for taping, describes how orthotics can accelerate an injured patient's return to competition. Chapter 3 provides an overview of the knee and describes the instabilities associated with ligament injury, as well as the role of preventive, rehabilitative, and functional bracing in injury management. Chapter 4 concerns the treatment of hip, thigh, and pelvic injuries, and chapter 5 moves on to the anatomy and injury mechanisms for the shoulder and arm. Chapter 6 presents the techniques available to the clinician when treating the elbow and forearm. Chapter 7 serves a similar purpose for wrist and hand injuries while also presenting the method for splinting tendon ruptures in the fingers.

KEY FEATURES

This four-color book provides state-of-the-art illustrations of anatomy and injury mechanisms. The quality of the photography is unsurpassed, and in the photographs the edges of the tape have been darkened for easier visualization of the taping patterns. Key palpation landmarks have also been identified and illustrated.

As with all health professions, evidence-based approaches to athletic training clinical practice are crucial to the effective delivery of health care. Research being conducted by people such as Carrie Docherty is contributing to the body of knowledge on taping and bracing. The extensive bibliography at the end of the book exemplifies this growing body of knowledge and is provided as a reference for students, clinicians, and researchers.

UPDATES

While the sound structure, organization, and key features of the third edition have been retained for this fourth edition, several updates have been made to the text. Most notably, Ian McLeod has joined as a coauthor for this fourth edition to present the application guidelines for casting and splinting and to illustrate several techniques throughout the book. Chapter 1 contains new information on casting and splinting in general, as well as application guidelines and precautions. Additionally, Carrie Docherty has joined us as a special contributor to chapter 1 to provide information explaining the importance of evidence-based practice for the techniques presented in the book. Finally, 20 new casting and splinting techniques are presented for Achilles tendon ruptures and common fractures of the foot, ankle, elbow, wrist, and hand.

INSTRUCTOR AND STUDENT RESOURCES

In addition to the text updates just discussed, the fourth edition of *Athletic Taping, Bracing, and Casting* also includes three new resources. An image bank includes all of the photos and illustrations from the text, and instructors can use these images to create handouts, illustrate a PowerPoint presentation, or create other learning aids for their students. Additionally, ready-made chapter quizzes that help assess student comprehension of the main concepts of each chapter are provided to instructors.

The web resource provides students with 56 competency checklists and 47 video clips, which help to illustrate the concepts being discussed in the text. The checklists detail the main steps an athletic training student must demonstrate to show competency in 56 different casting, splinting, and taping procedures, and instructors can use them during practical tests to ensure students are mastering the most important and useful casting, splinting, and taping procedures they will encounter in their athletic training careers.

When a video clip is available on the web resource, you will see an icon that looks like this:

These ancillaries can be accessed by visiting www.HumanKinetics.com/Athletic TapingBracingAndCasting. If you purchased a new print book, follow the directions included on the orange-framed page at the front of your book to access the web resource. That page includes access steps and the unique key code that you'll need the first time you visit the *Athletic Taping, Bracing, and Casting* website. If you purchased an ebook from HumanKinetics.com, follow the access instructions that were emailed to you following your purchase.

FINAL COMMENTS

Good luck as you embark on your journey into this exciting area of athletic training. The clinician skilled in the art and science of athletic taping, bracing, and casting quickly earns a patient's confidence. But becoming proficient at these skills is a challenge, and you should realize that achieving a high level of proficiency comes only after many hours—even years—of practice. Always visualize the underlying anatomy that you will be supporting and the mechanism of injury that you seek to prevent. You may feel frustration as you attempt to master these skills, but with concentration and practice, you can become highly adept at athletic taping, bracing, casting, and splinting.

Acknowledgments

We are indebted to many people for the roles they played in the publication of *Athletic Taping, Bracing, and Casting, Fourth Edition*. At Human Kinetics, the support of senior acquisitions editor Josh Stone, the expertise of developmental and managing editor Carly O'Connor, and the talent of video producer Gregg Henness and book designer Dawn Sills enabled the production of a much improved product. Thanks also to permissions manager Dalene Reeder.

We also want to extend our continued thanks to Primal Pictures, Ltd., for the use of the state-of-the art anatomy graphics and to Johnson & Johnson for providing the supplies used in many of the taping and wrapping procedures shown throughout the book. The supplies for the strapping tape and elastic kinesiology tape techniques used in the photos and videos were provided by Sammons Preston. Supplies for the casting and splinting techniques were provided by the Arizona Sports Medicine Center and the A.T. Still University Athletic Training Program.

Mariah Montoya and Alex Boron-Magulick joined previous models Abraham Jones, Aisei Mitsuhashi-Acs, Jatin Ambegaonkar, Kimberly Herndon, Tony Kulas, and Yohei Shimokochi as the enthusiastic models for the book.

Kip Smith served as a consultant for the photo shoot for the previous editions of this book, and he helped to illustrate several of the procedures in the book. Anne Keil contributed the text and illustrations for the strapping tape and kinesiology tape procedures. We are grateful to Kip and Anne for sharing their expertise.

Carrie Docherty, a leading researcher on the proper assessment and prevention of ankle instability, provided the new material related to evidence-based practice. She also contributed to the comprehensive bibliography found at the end of the book. We appreciate Carrie's willingness to be a contributor to the fourth edition.

CHAPTER 1

Introduction to Taping, Bracing, Casting, and Splinting

The National Athletic Trainers' Association's *Athletic Training Education Competencies, Fifth Edition*, has identified eight content areas to reflect athletic training clinical practice. An additional area—Clinical Integration Proficiencies (CIP)—reflects clinical practice and demonstrates the global nature of the Proficiencies. To become competent athletic trainers, students should master the knowledge, skills, and clinical abilities integral to each of the content areas listed in the sidebar Athletic Training Education Competencies. The knowledge, physical skills, and attitudes toward patients and the sports or physical activities in which they are engaged are also necessary for the application of tape and braces.

ANATOMY AS THE FOUNDATION TO TAPING, BRACING, CASTING, AND SPLINTING

A sound understanding of **human anatomy** is necessary for mastering the art and science of taping, bracing, and casting. You must understand the anatomical structures that you are attempting to support with the application of tape, a brace, a cast, or a splint. Anyone can learn the psychomotor skills required to tape or cast (the art), but you must also understand the link between the anatomical structure, the mechanism of injury, and the purpose for which tape or a cast is applied, such as immobilization, restriction of motion, or support of a ligament or muscle (the science). This book illustrates the most pertinent anatomical structures and mechanisms of injury for each of the body parts that you will learn to support with tape, a brace, a cast, or a splint. You should also be able to identify and palpate these anatomical structures through your understanding of **surface anatomy**. You will find a list of the key palpation landmarks in each chapter of the book.

Athletic Training Education Competencies

Evidence-based practice (EBP)

Prevention and health promotion (PHP)

Clinical examination and diagnosis (CE)

Acute care of injuries and illnesses (AC)

Therapeutic interventions (TI)

Psychosocial strategies and referral (PS)

Health care administration (HA)

Professional development and responsibility (PD)

Clinical Integration Proficiencies (CIP)

National Athletic Trainers' Association, *Athletic Training Education Competencies,* 5E (online), http://www.nata.org/sites/default/files/5th-Edition-Competencies-2011-PDF-Version.pdf

You will also need to learn and adopt the use of anatomical terminology in describing the position, planes, direction, and movement of the body. The **anatomical position** is the reference point for use of this terminology. The median plane bisects the body into right and left halves, and any plane parallel to the median plane is a sagittal plane. The coronal plane bisects the body into anterior (toward the front) and posterior (toward the back) portions. The transverse (axial) plane divides the body into superior (upper) and inferior (lower) parts.

In describing the limbs, proximal (closer to) and distal (farther from) identify structures nearer to or farther from the attachment of the limb to the torso. The position of the paired bones of the extremities is often used to describe anatomical location. For example, the thumb is on the radial side of the forearm, and the great toe is on the tibial side of the lower extremity. Palmar and plantar are used to describe the anterior surfaces of the hand and foot, respectively, and dorsal describes the other side in both the hand and foot.

Specific terms also describe movements of the body. Flexion means bending in a direction that usually reduces the angle of a joint, and extension is the opposite movement. Abduction means movement away from the midline, and adduction is the opposite motion. Rotation is movement of a bone around its long axis, and it occurs in the medial (inward) or lateral (outward) direction. Joint-specific terms describe movements at the forearm and foot. Supination and pronation describe

Anatomical Position

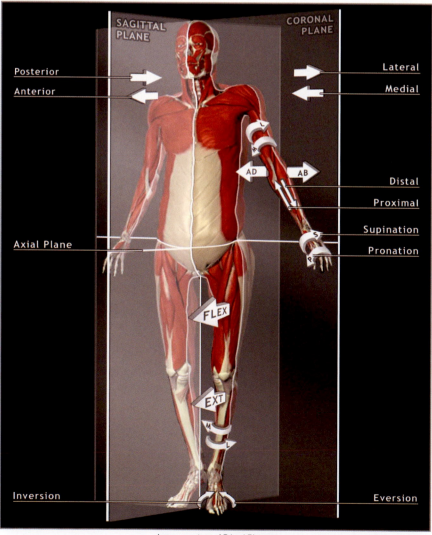

Image courtesy of Primal Pictures

movement of the forearm to position the palm up and down, respectively (with the elbow at 90° of flexion). Inversion and eversion move the sole of the foot inward or outward, respectively. Circumduction is a combination of movements at joints that permits flexion, abduction, extension, and adduction.

The taping, wrapping, bracing and casting techniques that you will learn in this book are designed to support and protect injuries to the bones, ligaments, tendons, muscles, nerves, and joints of the body. Some of the more common injuries for which you will apply tape, wraps, casts, and splints are illustrated throughout the text.

Knee Joint

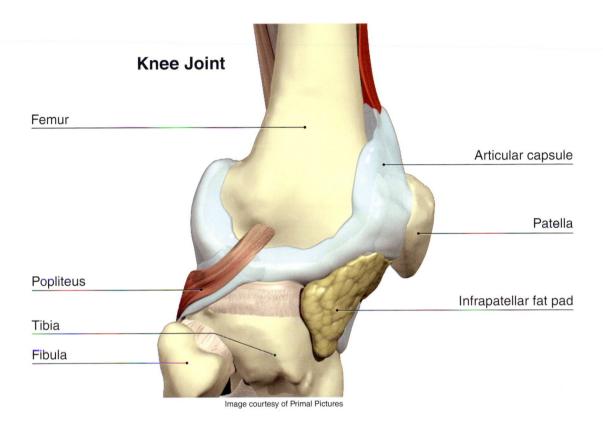

Image courtesy of Primal Pictures

Shoulder Complex

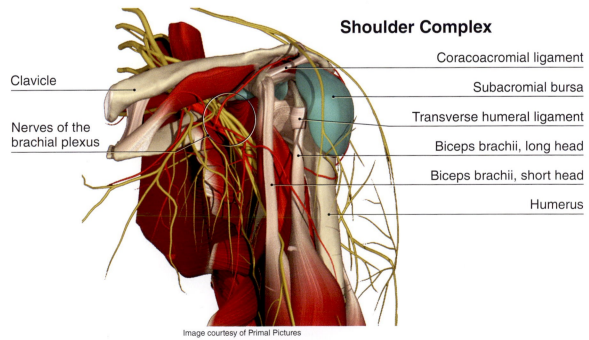

Image courtesy of Primal Pictures

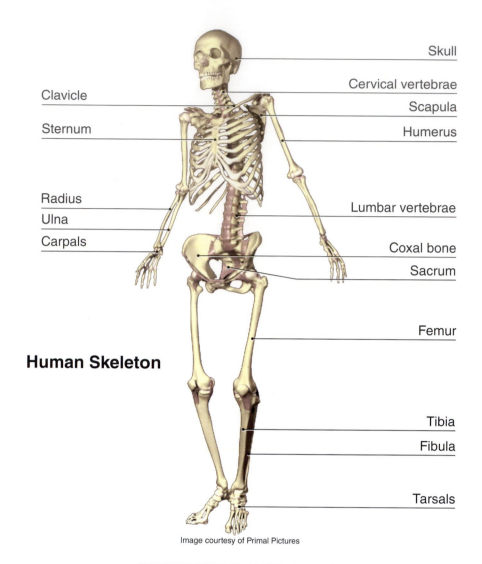

Human Skeleton

- Skull
- Cervical vertebrae
- Scapula
- Humerus
- Clavicle
- Sternum
- Radius
- Ulna
- Carpals
- Lumbar vertebrae
- Coxal bone
- Sacrum
- Femur
- Tibia
- Fibula
- Tarsals

Image courtesy of Primal Pictures

EVIDENCE-BASED PRACTICE OF TAPING, BRACING, CASTING, AND SPLINTING

Over the years, evidence-based practice (EBP) has been an integral part of the decision making process when interacting with athletes and patients. A common definition of EBP is the integration of best research evidence along with clinician expertise and patient needs to inform clinical decisions. One area in which clinicians spend a significant amount of time (and money) is through taping, bracing, and splinting techniques. Therefore, it is critically important that these decisions are based on this EBP model. The most recent edition of the Athletic Training Education Competencies recommends a five-step approach when employing evidence-based practice:

1. Creating a clinically relevant question
2. Searching for the best evidence
3. Critically analyzing the evidence
4. Integrating the appraisal with personal clinical expertise and the patients' preferences
5. Evaluating the performance or outcomes of the actions

Therefore, prior to applying any taping, bracing, or casting technique, or combination of techniques, the purpose of the application should be identified. For many of these techniques the purpose is to prevent a future injury from occurring, but the method used for this prevention can vary. Injuries can be prevented through such methods as restricting range of motion, enhancing proprioception, and improving joint alignment.

The following is an example of how a clinician would utilize the five-step approach in her or his evidence-based practice:

1. "Does the application of ankle bracing reduce the risk of ankle injury?"
2. Table 1.1 outlines the relevant research pertaining to the preceding question.
3. While all of the studies in table 1.1 were randomized control trials and could be classified as "good" quality evidence, there are still other things to consider, such as: How long ago was the study conducted? What type of brace was used? What are the characteristics of the participants? How many participants were included? How long did they follow the participants?
4. Based on this information, the clinician could conclude that lace-up ankle bracing can be effective in preventing ankle sprains in people with a history of ankle injuries. However, it is unclear whether ankle braces are effective in preventing ankle sprains in people without a history of ankle injuries. Then the clinician would consider his or her own ability to provide a brace for the patient as well as the patient's ability to properly wear it. The clinician would also review the patient's history of previous ankle injuries as well as any considerations related to the patient's sport or activity or attitude toward bracing.
5. Based on the answer to all of these questions, the clinician would come to an evidence-based conclusion. Finally, the clinician should track the patient's injury status at 6 and 12 months and 2 years after treatment in an effort to continually provide additional evidence to the model.

Table 1.1 Relevant Published Research to Answer the Question, "Does the Application of Ankle Bracing Reduce the Risk of Ankle Injury?"

Title	Year	Design	Findings
McGuine TA, Brooks A, Hetzel S. The effect of lace-up ankle braces on injury rates in high school basketball players. *Am J Sports Med.* 2011:39(9):1840-1848.	2011	Randomized control trial Two groups (brace and no brace)	• Ankle injury incidence rates were lower in the brace group for subjects both with and without a previous history of ankle injuries • Severity of ankle sprains did not differ between the groups
McGuine TA, Hetzel S, Wilson J, Brooks A. The effect of lace-up ankle braces on injury rates in high school football players. *Am J Sports Med.* 2012:40(1):49-57.	2012	Randomized control trial Two groups (brace and no brace)	• Ankle injury incidence rates were lower in the brace group for subjects both with and without a previous history of ankle injuries • Severity of ankle sprains did not differ between the groups
Sitler M, Ryan J, Wheeler B, et al. The efficacy of a semirigid ankle stabilizer to reduce acute ankle injuries in basketball: A randomized clinical study at West Point. *Am J Sports Med.* 1994;22(4):454-461.	1994	Randomized control trial Two groups (brace and no brace)	• Braces reduced the incidence of sprains in military cadets participating in intramural basketball teams • No difference in injury severity between the groups
Mohammadi F. Comparison of 3 preventive methods to reduce the recurrence of ankle inversion sprains in male soccer players. *Am J Sports Med.* 2007;35(6):922-926.	2007	Randomized control trial Four groups (brace, no brace, rehab 1, and rehab 2)	• Use of an ankle brace did not affect the number of ankle sprains compared to the control group • Very small sample
Surve I, Schwellnus MP, Noakes T, Lombard C. A fivefold reduction in the incidence of recurrent ankle sprains in soccer players using Sport-Stirrup orthosis. *Am J Sports Med.*1994;22(5):601-606.	1994	Randomized control trial Two groups (brace and no brace)	• Ankle brace is effective in reducing the incidence of ankle injuries in people with a history of ankle sprains • Ankle brace had no effect on people with no history of ankle sprains

EBP is only effective when relevant, high-quality studies have been conducted and published. In reviewing the literature of the taping techniques included in this textbook, it became clear that limited research is available for many of these techniques. Significant work has been done in the foot and ankle, but as you move up the kinetic chain, research resources become limited. Additional research should be conducted, particularly in the upper extremity. Research has been completed investigating techniques using specialized tape, such as kinesiology and rigid strapping tape, but even with these techniques the studies often result in conflicting conclusions.

ROLE OF TAPING, BRACING, CASTING, AND SPLINTING

Although the National Athletic Trainers' Association's structure for the domains of athletic training lists taping as only one of several abilities necessary for athletic trainers to function effectively, it is one of the most important, and most visible, skills. You can quickly earn a patient's confidence through proficient application of athletic tape. Learning to master this task, however, will be both rewarding and frustrating. As with any psychomotor skill, taping requires a great deal of practice before the clinician achieves excellence.

Athletic taping, bracing, casting, and splinting can prevent injury or facilitate an injured patient's return to competition. In general, the tape should limit abnormal or excessive movement of a **sprained** joint while also providing support to the muscle that the sprain has compromised. Many clinicians attribute the value of taping to the enhanced proprioceptive feedback that the tape provides the patient during performance. For example, patients who have injured the anterior cruciate ligament and suffer from rotary instability in the knee may receive sensory cues from the brace before it limits rotary movement. This early **proprioceptive** feedback may enable the patient subconsciously to contract the muscles that control rotary instability. Similarly, patients involved in volleyball and basketball may receive sensory cues from a taped ankle that experiences inversion while airborne. Tape, in this instance, can be more effective in providing proprioceptive feedback than in actually limiting excessive inversion.

Regardless of how tape and braces work, they should not substitute for exercise. Routine taping of the ankle in the absence of preactivity exercise provides the patient with substandard health care. For this reason, taping should work in conjunction with stretching and strengthening techniques. As a matter of policy, you should tape or brace only those patients willing to comply with your requests to attain and maintain optimal joint range of motion and muscle strength.

Athletic Training Education Competencies
Pertinent to Athletic Taping, Bracing, Casting, and Splinting

Prevention and Health Promotion

► Protective equipment and prophylactic procedures: Apply preventive taping and wrapping procedures, splints, braces, and other special protective devices.

Therapeutic Interventions

► Physical rehabilitation and therapeutic modalities: Fabricate and apply taping, wrapping, supportive, and protective devices to facilitate return to function.

Clinical Integration Proficiencies

► Prevention and health promotion: Select, apply, evaluate, and modify appropriate standard protective equipment, taping, wrapping, bracing, padding, and other custom devices for the patient in order to prevent or minimize the risk of injury to the head, torso, spine, and extremities for safe participation in sport or other physical activity.

In contrast to athletic taping, where a primary goal is to limit abnormal or excessive movement, splinting and casting are commonly utilized when a patient sustains an injury that requires immobilization for a specified duration of time. The primary goals of immobilization include prevention of further soft-tissue and bony injury, pain reduction, maintenance of fracture alignment, and promotion of healing. When properly applied, the rigid nature of splinting and casting materials allows the immobilization of joints and stabilization of anatomic structures such as ligaments, tendons, and bones. The benefit of the added protection does carry the risk of muscle atrophy (strength loss) and joint stiffness (range of motion loss), which correlate directly to the length of immobilization.

Splinting utilizes a non-circumferential rigid material, most commonly fiberglass, held in place by an elastic wrap to immobilize an injured area (see figure 1.1). Since the splint does not fully envelope the injured area with rigid material, splinting can accommodate for post-traumatic swelling, making it the preferred method of immobilization for acute injuries. Splints are easier to apply and can be applied more quickly than casts, which is advantageous when treating acute injuries, especially if the injured area is unstable. Because splints are held in place by an elastic wrap, clinicians can easily remove them to inspect the skin, which is important if there is a skin wound (e.g., cut or abrasion) or surgical incision that is covered by the splinting materials. If indicated, a splint can be removed in order to administer therapy for a soft-tissue injury. While the ability for clinicians to remove the splint to evaluate and treat the injured area is advantageous, one concern with splints is that patients are also able to remove the splint on their own. Educating the patient on the importance of keeping the injured area immobilized and the potential complications associated with removing the splint can significantly improve compliance. Another disadvantage of splinting is that because the rigid support is non-circumferential it does not offer as much stability as casting.

In contrast to splinting, casting involves applying fiberglass or plaster circumferentially around the injured area to create a more rigid support that is much stronger than a splint (see figure 1.2). Because casts are stronger, they provide superior stability and protection, and therefore are the preferred method of long-term immobilization for fractures. The

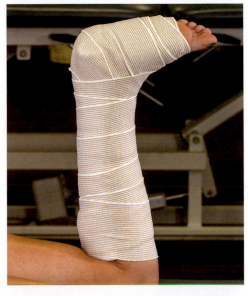

Figure 1.1 Posterior ankle splint immobilizing the ankle.

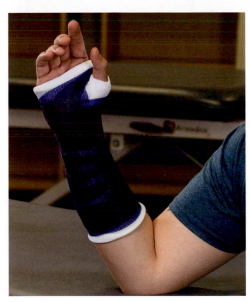

Figure 1.2 Fiberglass short arm cast immobilizing the wrist.

increased strength of the cast comes at a cost in the form of extra materials, making casts heavier, and therefore more burdensome, than splints. Casts are also more difficult and time-consuming to apply. One concern with casting too soon after the injury is that casts are unable to expand and therefore cannot accommodate swelling, which is why it is best to wait to apply a cast until the post-traumatic swelling has resolved.

Factors that determine whether it would be best to use a splint or cast to protect the area include the injury acuity, body part involved, type of injury, and timeframe for healing. It is common to use splints for acute injuries in which there is the potential for post-traumatic swelling, soft-tissue injuries that require short term (<2 weeks) immobilization, stable simple fractures, or injuries that require stabilization prior to definitive treatment (e.g., immobilizing unstable or complex fracture pending **surgical fixation**). Once post-traumatic swelling has resolved, casts are preferred for definitive fracture care, especially in cases that involve unstable or complex fractures. A patient's risk for complications also factors into deciding if it would be best to utilize a splint or a cast. For example, regardless of the underlying injury (e.g., simple fracture versus complex fracture) it is a contraindication to apply a cast over an open wound due to the risk of developing an infection. On the other hand, if you are concerned that a patient may not comply with the recommendation to keep a splint on at all times, it may be best to immobilize the area with a cast.

As with any therapeutic intervention, prior to applying a splint or cast the clinician should weigh the risks and benefits to ensure that benefits of immobilizing the injured area outweigh the potential complications that could arise with immobilizing the injured area. Complications that can occur with splinting or casting include the following:

- Joint stiffness and active and passive range of motion loss
- Muscle atrophy and decrease in muscle strength
- Increased risk of venous thromboembolism (blood clot)
- Vascular compromise
- Skin irritation and skin breakdown
- Pressure sores and ulcers
- Thermal injury and burns
- Nerve injury
- Compartment syndrome
- Complex regional pain syndrome
- Chronic pain
- Fracture non-union

Risk factors that influence the potential for complications during a period of immobilization with a splint or cast are categorized as uncontrollable and controllable. Uncontrollable risk factors include age of the patient, previous injuries, comorbid conditions (e.g., diabetes mellitus increases risk of neurovascular complication), type of injury, and severity of injury. Controllable risk factors include the method of immobilization, the type of material used, the quality of the splint or cast, and the duration of immobilization.

APPARATUS OF TAPING AND BRACING

A variety of tools are needed to cover the different taping and bracing needs of injured patients. These include elastic (figure 1.3) or nonelastic (figure 1.4) athletic tape, cloth, wraps, and braces. Manufacturers produce and market athletic tape in many sizes and textures.

Purposes of Taping and Bracing

▶ Support the ligaments and capsule of unstable joints by limiting excessive or abnormal anatomical movement.
▶ Enhance proprioceptive feedback from the limb or joint.
▶ Support injuries to the muscle–tendon units by compressing and limiting movement.
▶ Secure protective pads, dressings, and splints.

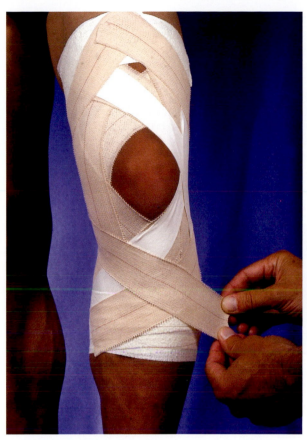

Figure 1.3   Application of elastic tape to support the knee.

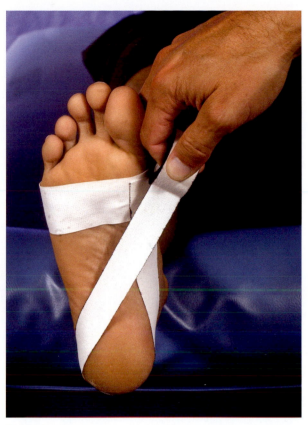

Figure 1.4   Application of nonelastic tape to support the arch.

Nonelastic Tape and Cloth

Use nonelastic tape to provide optimal joint support and to restrict abnormal or excessive joint motion. For example, nonelastic white tape applied directly to the ankle can prevent excessive inversion.

Nonelastic white tape is normally porous and is available in 15-yard (13.7 m) rolls with widths of 1, 1.5, or 2 inches (2.5, 3.8, or 5.1 cm). The size of the patient, the anatomical site, and the preference of the athletic trainer will dictate which width to use.

Although nonelastic tape provides the best support, it has the disadvantage of being the most difficult to use. When applying nonelastic white tape you will find that the contours of the body can easily cause the tape to wrinkle. You will need a great deal of practice to master the smooth and efficient application of nonelastic tape.

Nonelastic cloth wraps can provide support independently or in combination with white tape (figure 1.5). Cloth wraps, although not as convenient as tape, provide acceptable support at considerable cost savings; consider them if your budgetary resources are limited.

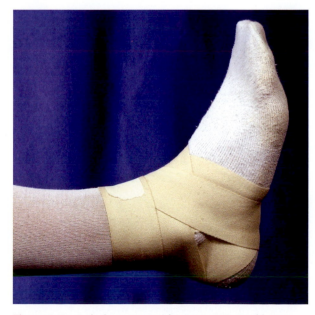

Figure 1.5   A cloth wrap provides inexpensive ankle support. The cloth wrap is also an excellent way to practice the figure-eight and heel-lock techniques presented in chapter 2.

Elastic Tape and Wraps

Apply elastic tape or wraps to support body parts that, unlike most joints, require great freedom of movement. For example, when it is necessary to support the hamstrings muscle group by encircling the thigh, use elastic tape to permit normal muscle contraction without restricting blood flow. Elastic tape and wraps will also secure protective pads to the body (figure 1.6). A patient with thigh, hip, or shoulder **contusions** often requires this extra protection; we will discuss the technique further in chapters 4 and 5.

Elastic wraps prove especially useful when applying compression to an area that has suffered an **acute injury**. Compression, frequently combined with ice, helps control the swelling that accompanies soft-tissue injuries (figure 1.7).

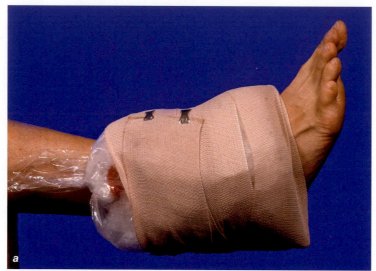

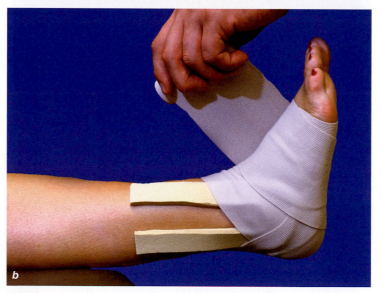

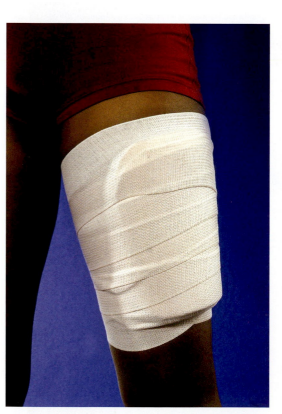

Figure 1.6   An elastic wrap to secure a protective pad to the anterior thigh. The metal clips used to fasten an elastic wrap should be covered with tape or removed for participation.

Figure 1.7   (a) Elastic wrap to secure an ice bag to the ankle. Apply the ice directly to the skin for no longer than 20 minutes per hour. (b) The elastic wrap can also be used in combination with a horseshoe pad to apply compression to an acutely sprained ankle.

When treating patients with this technique, you should always advise them about the potential risks of applying elastic wraps to acute injuries that will, inevitably, swell. In particular, you should warn the patients to watch for signs of restricted circulation by monitoring the color of fingernail or toenail beds. A dark blue appearance in a nail bed indicates impaired circulation. If the elastic wrap is necessary, be certain to remind the patient to elevate the injured joint and apply the wrap loosely if used at night.

Elastic tape, like nonelastic tape, comes in textures and widths for every body part. Elastic tape can be 1, 2, 3, or 4 inches (2.5, 5.1, 7.6, or 10.2 cm) wide. Elastic wraps may have widths of 2, 3, 4, or 6 inches (5.1, 7.6, 10.2. or 15.2 cm); they are also available in double lengths to accommodate large body areas, such as the hip and trunk. Elastic wrap quality varies. Because you reuse elastic wraps, unlike tape, you could save money by buying the better, often more expensive, product. The cheaper, low-quality wraps do not work well for continued reapplication.

Protective Devices in Combination With Tape and Wraps

Protective splints and pads are frequently used to limit motion, protect a body part, or dissipate forces away from the injured area. Athletic tape and wraps can often be used to hold the protective splints and pads in place. The protective materials include foam, felt, thermoplastics, thermofoams, and other materials such as fiberglass, silicone rubber, and neoprene. The book will provide selected examples of these protective materials and the use of tape and wraps to hold them in place.

Athletic Braces

Braces prevent injury to healthy joints and support unstable joints. A variety of braces is available in the athletic marketplace. In fact, you can find a brace for every joint of the body; although, for athletic purposes, you will most commonly need to apply braces for the ankle, knee, shoulder, elbow, and wrist. We will not supply a comprehensive review of braces; we will focus, instead, on those used to treat common ligament injuries in the ankle and knee and overuse injuries in the elbow and wrist. In addition, we provide photos for ankle, knee, wrist, elbow, and shoulder braces in their respective chapters.

Braces can supplement or replace athletic tape. Some braces, such as those for the ankle, can save money because, unlike athletic tape, they are reusable. Braces, however, can be expensive. Functional knee braces, for example, cost from $500 to $700.

Rigid Strapping Tape and Elastic Kinesiology Tape

The effectiveness of traditional athletic tape tends to decrease during physical activity. Alternatives to traditional athletic tape are rigid strapping tape and elastic kinesiology tape.

Rigid Strapping Tape

Underwrap tape plus rigid strapping tape (figure 1.8) adheres better than traditional athletic tape and allows patients to withstand activity longer. Rigid strapping tapes have only a 30% stretch from the time of initial application and are therefore more useful for creating a bracing type of support to the area. This lack of stretch in the tape is especially important if the person is engaged in physical activity and is relying on stability gained from the tape. A tape underwrap is usually applied before the rigid tape is applied. The therapeutic effects of strapping tape include stabilizing joints, improving joint movement and tolerance to loading, changing and controlling posture or small deformities, aiding in assessment for use of orthotics, facilitating muscle activity and control, inhibiting muscle activity, reducing pain by unloading structures, increasing motor neuron excitability, increasing joint torque, and enhancing proprioception. (For more information on using rigid strapping tape, see Keil, 2012.)

Elastic Kinesiology Tape

The other form of therapeutic taping involves elastic kinesiology tape, such as Kinesio Tape (figure 1.9), which has elasticity up to 140% of the tape's original length. This elastic tape allows full joint motion and aids lymphatic flow. Elastic kinesiology tape is latex free and water resistant. Despite its popularity, evidence for the effectiveness of kinesiology taping as the only treatment technique for an injury is limited, conflicting, and lacking in quality. Kinesiology taping is effective in reducing pain, increasing range of motion, and changing electromyographic (EMG) activity. However, these conditions are true only when used in conjunction with other physical therapy techniques such as manual therapy and exercise in people with neurological problems such as stroke or cerebral palsy or in people with orthopedic injuries. Benefits of kinesiology taping include joint support and unloading, stretching fascial tightness, decreasing lymphatic congestion (by stimulating lymph flow when the taping is directed toward the lymph collectors in the neck, axilla, medial elbow, dorsum of the wrist, spine, sacrum, groin, medial knee, and Achilles areas), normalizing muscle function by assisting muscle facilitation (decreasing fatigue) and inhibition (decreasing hypertonicity and cramping), increasing proprioceptive input, increasing joint range of motion, and decreasing pain.

Application Guidelines for Strap Taping and Kinesiology Taping

First, as with athletic taping, obtain an accurate assessment of the cause or contribution to the symptoms. This is especially important considering the activity that the patient

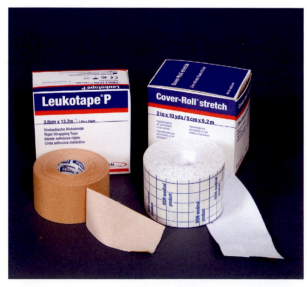

Figure 1.8   Leukotape strapping tape and Cover-Roll underwrap.

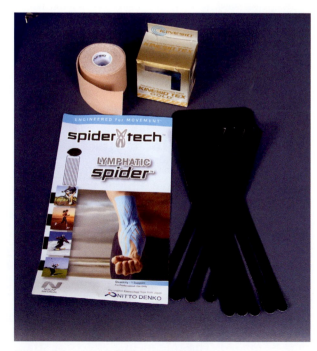

Figure 1.9   Kinesio Tape and Spidertech.

wishes to perform. Taping is used as an adjunct to other treatment options, including exercising for muscle imbalances, stretching tight muscles, postural retraining, biomechanically evaluating form during the aggravating activity, and using manual therapy to address joint restrictions. A good knowledge of anatomy and biomechanics is imperative in choosing the most beneficial type of tape and the most appropriate technique, depending on the goal of the taping application.

Many athletic taping techniques can be modified (e.g., using less tape) when applying strapping tape. Taping is a creative process as long as the precautions are kept in mind and the patient's pain or symptoms have decreased once the tape is applied. Taping alone will not suffice in the assessment and treatment of injuries; a thorough evaluation by a qualified health professional is an essential first step in determining appropriate treatment options.

Precautions for Strap Taping and Kinesiology Taping

There are a few differences in precautions related to strapping tape and kinesiology tape compared to athletic tape:

1. *Allergy to latex or adhesives.* Cover-Roll (underwrap tape product) does not contain latex, whereas Leukotape and other brands of strapping tape do. Kinesiology tape is latex free and is applied directly to the skin. Strap taping techniques can be applied to people with allergies to latex, usually without problems, but the strapping tape should *not* come in direct contact with the skin. If there is a skin allergy or sensitivity to either latex or adhesives, a red raised rash will appear directly under the tape and may be very itchy. Allergy will occur usually within the first 24 hours but could appear up to 10 days after application. It is common for the skin to be red when the tape is removed, especially if it has been on the skin for a long time. This usually fades within a few minutes to a few hours. Cortisone or other topical anti-inflammatory cream can be used if skin is irritated. Calamine lotion or liquid antacid can also be helpful when spread over the affected skin areas; otherwise, a skin protectant can be used before application.

2. *Friction rub or blistering.* This occurs in areas where a forceful pull or anchor is applied with strapping tape. Skin can break down and tear in certain areas of tension or excessive movement (most commonly seen around the anterior or medial knee). Skin in this area will toughen with time and not be as susceptible to breakdown.

3. *Taping technique that limits joint range of motion.* When using strapping tape, be aware of the range of motion that the patient requires to perform his or her activity so that when the area is taped, the joint mobility is not limited and performance is not inhibited. Also make sure the tape is not causing excessive pull, which can lead to a friction rub or blistering.

4. *Impaired circulation distal to taping.* When taping (especially when using rigid tape) completely around a joint (elbow, knee, ankle, wrist), ensure that the tape isn't so tight that it impairs circulation to the area distal to the tape. This can impede venous return and cause swelling in the area (e.g., hand or foot) as well as more serious complications.

5. *Fragile skin.* Use caution when taping persons with delicate skin (e.g., elderly, children, patients with connective tissue disorders, those with diabetes who are prone to skin breakdown), taping over open or scabbed wounds, or taping after recent surgery (i.e., on scars that have not fully closed). It is possible to tape over a plastic bandage covering an open wound or scab and have patients wear the tape for shorter periods so that the wound status can be checked. A patient who has problems with skin integrity can wear a small test strip of underwrap tape on the skin for a couple of days to see how it is tolerated.

Application of Strapping Tape

1. Prepare the skin area to be taped. Make sure it is shaved, clean (wipe with rubbing alcohol if skin appears dirty or oily), and free of residual adhesive from prior taping (use adhesive remover). Remove clothing that impairs access to the area to be taped.

2. Position the patient so he or she is in the best neutral anatomical position during the taping, ensuring that you have easy access to the body part you will be taping. Some techniques require two clinicians for optimal effectiveness.

3. Measure and cut strips of underwrap and apply them with enough coverage so the strapping tape will not contact skin (except in the case of taping the foot, where underwrap is optional).

4. Cut or tear strips of strapping tape and apply them with adequate tension in the direction of pull desired to create some wrinkling in the underwrap and sometimes wrinkling or gathering of the skin (figure 1.10).

5. Assess the integrity of the tape by taking the joint through some range of motion necessary for the activity the patient will perform (e.g., have the patient bend and straighten the knee if the knee was taped or walk if the foot was taped). You might need to apply pressure to the ends of the tape if the edges start to pull loose, or you can add anchor strips of underwrap to the end of the taping strips to secure them (figure 1.11).

6. Assess the completed taping for change in symptoms or pain control. Tape should quickly do its job and decrease pain in the area when the patient moves in a way that previously was causing pain. Sometimes changing the angle or force of pull with strapping tape may be necessary. If tape does not improve symptoms or causes pain in another area, it should be removed.

7. Give the patient instruction on wear time. With strapping tape, depending on the integrity of the tape and skin tolerance, tape can be worn 2 to 7 days through showers and sweating, and it should remain intact. Swimming or excessive exposure to water will decrease adherence time. Oily or very sweaty skin will also decrease adherence time, especially on the foot. Tape edges will become ragged first and then start to peel off. When there is no longer enough tension, or symptoms start to return, then it is time to remove the tape. The patient needs to wear the tape until the muscles have become strong enough to support the area needed for the activity, and the muscles need to have the endurance to maintain the position for the desired time. Typically, if symptoms are acute, the patient will wear the tape for 3 to 5 days during normal activity. Once pain has diminished, the patient can slowly incorporate the sport activity into the routine, applying tape only for aggressive activities. Most of the time, when muscle strength and endurance have improved, the patient won't need to use tape during all activities. The patient will, however, need to use good biomechanics forever.

8. When the tape needs to be removed, start peeling the tape off at an edge of the underwrap and peel slowly so as not to tear the skin. Removal is easiest when the tape or skin is wet, such as after a shower, bath, or swimming.

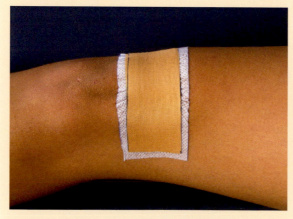

Figure 1.10 Tension applied to strapping tape.

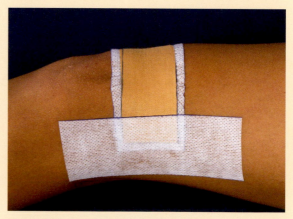

Figure 1.11 Anchor strips of underwrap.

Application of Kinesiology Tape

1. Apply the tape 20 minutes to 1 hour before activity to ensure best adhesion, or use tape adherent if applying during an activity. Use water-resistant tape if applying to sweaty areas or to hands and feet. Kinesiology tape is water resistant starting 1 hour after application.

2. Start and end the tape strips without tension. Cut ends of the tape round to prevent rolling of tape corners. Tape will bunch the skin and be convoluted, creating pressure pocket and vacuum effects. Start and end pieces of tape on the skin, not over another piece of tape. Peel off 1 to 2 inches (2.5-5 cm) of paper backing or make a small tear in the backing to help remove it. Adhere it to the skin, then take the joint through its full range of motion and press the rest of the strip of tape to the skin. Avoid excessive stretching of tape before application. Avoid layering more than three pieces of tape over one area because tape will not adhere well.

3. There are four common ways to cut the tape. The I-cut (figure 1.12*a*) is used on all muscles and is applied directly over the affected muscle or to cross a joint for increased stability and for acute muscle injury. The Y-cut (figure 1.12*b*) is the most common technique used to surround muscles and relax spasms or increase strength of weak muscles and increase lymph flow. The X-cut (figure 1.12*c*) stabilizes the joint relative to the targeted muscle. The fan cut (figure 1.12*d*) is for edema reduction when the point that you want lymph to drain toward is the base of the fan.

   ▶ To alleviate spasms, tape from muscle **insertion** to origin with the muscle stretched (e.g., when taping the calf, dorsiflex the ankle).

   ▶ To treat weak muscles, tape from muscle origin to insertion while elongating the opposing muscle (e.g., stretch the pectoralis muscle if applying a technique to affect the upper trapezius or posterior deltoid). This application of tape will bunch the skin.

   ▶ To assist with bruising, edema, or circulation problems, apply little or no tension. To affect muscle, apply tape with light to moderate tension. To help stabilize joints or ligaments, apply the most tension.

4. After application, rub tape to activate the heat-sensitive adhesive. When tape gets wet (e.g., after showering), pat it dry with a towel or use a hair dryer to dry it. (Caution: Excessive heat from a dryer makes the tape more difficult to remove.) There is usually a 3- to 10-day wear time. If the tape edges lift, they can be trimmed off if tape is otherwise intact.

5. To remove the tape, pull it off in the direction of hair growth while holding down the skin around it. For a more comfortable removal, saturate the tape with baby oil, vegetable oil, or a tape removal product for 15 to 20 minutes before removal.

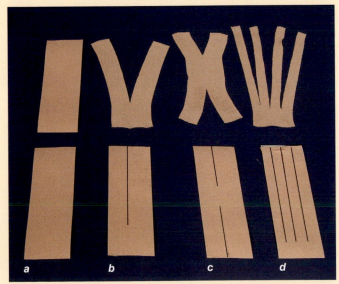

Figure 1.12 Common cuts to kinesiology tape: *(a)* I-cut, *(b)* Y-cut, *(c)* X-cut, and *(d)* fan cut. The lines drawn on the solid pieces of tape on the bottom row show where you would cut the tape to create the various kinesiology tape cuts.

APPARATUS OF SPLINTING AND CASTING

Fiberglass and plaster are the most commonly used materials to create rigid splints and casts. Most clinicians have migrated to using fiberglass because it is stronger, lighter, more breathable, and cleaner to apply than plaster. Additionally, once fiberglass has hardened it maintains its integrity whereas plaster begins to break down and lose its shape when it is wet. Plaster has a slower setting time and is more moldable, which makes it easier to apply and allows the clinician more time to apply the splint or cast. While novice clinicians consider the slower setting time an advantage, experienced clinicians deem it a hindrance.

A characteristic shared by both fiberglass and plaster is that the hardening of the material is due to an exothermic reaction. Exothermic reactions produce heat, and if applied incorrectly, a fiberglass splint or cast has the potential to cause first or second-degree burns. Exposure to water catalyzes the exothermic reaction, and the higher the water temperature, the more heat is available to cause the material to harden faster, which in turn increases the amount of heat produced. By using water that is at room temperature or cooler, you can reduce the risk of thermal injury.

Plaster is available in 1- to 6-inch (2.5-15 cm) wide rolls and as strips with white as the only color option. Fiberglass is available in 1- to 6-inch (2.5-15 cm) wide rolls with numerous color options available. Prefabricated plaster and fiberglass splints with or without padding are available in 3- to 6-inch (8-15 cm) wide rolls that are 15 feet (4.5 m) long or as individual prepackaged splints that range from 10 to 35 inches (25-89 cm) long. While the prefabricated splints are convenient, they can be very expensive.

Prior to applying a splint or cast, a protective barrier is applied to reduce the risk of skin irritation and skin breakdown. The first layer is composed of tubular stockinette (see figure 1.13a), which is a thin, sock-like material that has the ability to expand. Tubular stockinette is available in width sizes from 1 to 6 inches (2.5-15 cm). Smaller stockinette, 1 to 3 inches (2.5-8 cm), is used for the upper extremities, and larger

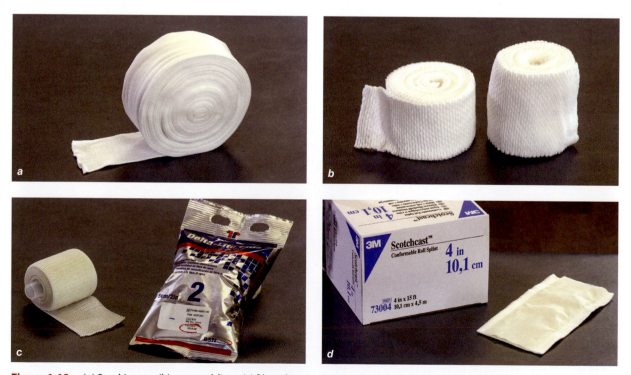

Figure 1.13   (a) Stockinette, (b) cast padding, (c) fiberglass casting tape, and (d) prefabricated fiberglass splint.

stockinette, 3 to 6 inches (8-15 cm), is used for the lower extremities. Cotton or synthetic cast padding (see figure 1.13*b*) composes the next layer and functions to protect against thermal injury when the splint or cast is initially applied, accommodating for small amounts of swelling and absorbing moisture to prevent maceration of the skin. Cast padding is available in width sizes from 1 to 6 inches (2.5-15 cm) and, similar to stockinette, the smaller sizes are used for the upper extremities and the larger sizes are used for the lower extremities. When applying cast padding, begin at the distal portion of the extremity and roll the padding circumferentially from distal to proximal, overlapping by 50%. This will provide two layers of cast padding; your goal is to have two to three layers of cast padding. You should apply extra padding over bony prominences and over the locations where the splint or cast begin and end. Be aware that excessive cast padding will compromise the ability of the splint or cast to adequately immobilize and protect the injured area. Splinting or casting material (see figure 1.13*c* and *d*) is then applied directly over the cast padding. The following is a list of items used in applying splints and casts.

- Plaster or fiberglass splinting and casting material
- Stockinette
- Cast padding
- Elastic wrap
- Casting gloves
- Casting scissors (best to have a pair dedicated to cutting fiberglass and a separate pair for cutting other materials)
- Water basin
- Protective barrier to prevent soiling of patient's clothing
- Blue disposable under pads (Chux pad)

KNOWING THE SPORT, PATIENT, AND INJURY

To become an effective athletic trainer, you must learn both anatomy and the **mechanisms of injury** and master the psychomotor tasks for appropriate athletic taping. In addition, you should understand the rules of the sport regarding taping, bracing, and casting and the needs of your individual patients.

Regulation of Taping, Bracing, and Casting in Sport

Most governing athletic associations regulate the degree of restriction you can provide through taping, bracing, and casting as well as the materials that you use to protect an injured part. They enforce these mandates because the application of tape can give the wearer an unfair advantage during competition, especially in sports such as wrestling. Protective devices and braces can also injure other participants. Most associations prohibit hard and inflexible materials unless you cover them with a soft, pliable padding.

Sport associations also regulate the management of athletic injuries during organized competition. Wrestling, for example, permits only a short time to treat an injured patient. Many other sports require you to remove the patient from competition, regardless of the severity of the injury. You must also follow universal precautions if the patient is bleeding, so you should become very familiar with these procedures. These and other rules affect how you evaluate an injured patient and apply a brace or tape. You should consult the guidelines of your appropriate governing organization, such as the National Collegiate Athletic Association or a state or regional high school athletic association.

Knowing the Patient

Some patients cannot perform with even a small degree of restricted movement, whereas others do quite well with a great deal of limitation. A significant amount of restriction on the hands and fingers of a football offensive or defensive lineman may not inhibit the patient's performance. In contrast, the same, or even a lesser, degree of restriction would dramatically compromise the dexterity of a quarterback or receiver. Taping a shot-putter's ankle requires you to use a technique different from the one you apply when supporting the ankle of a sprinter. These examples show that to master the art and science of taping, you must understand the different needs of your patients.

Examining and Treating the Injury

You must have a thorough mastery of injury assessment and rehabilitation to tape and brace effectively, including knowing when it is safe to return a patient to practice and competition.

Injury Assessment Protocol

- Obtain the patient's history relating to the mechanism of injury.
- Inspect the area for swelling and deformity.
- Palpate the part for abnormalities.
- Assess the active range of motion; that is, determine the patient's willingness and ability to move the part.
- Determine the passive range of motion; that is, while the patient relaxes, move the part through its maximum range of motion.
- Evaluate the resistive range of motion; that is, assess the patient's ability to contract the muscles about the part.
- Apply special tests to assess the integrity of the ligaments of the joint.
- Always compare your findings with the uninjured extremity!

Injury Examination

Under no circumstance should you tape, brace, cast, or splint a patient's injury without first knowing the injury mechanism and its underlying anatomical structure. By understanding the mechanism of injury you will be able to apply tape, a brace, a splint, or a cast in a manner that will help prevent further damage. To determine the injury mechanism and know whether the injury is acute or **chronic**, you must obtain a patient's history. Be systematic in your evaluation by using the information in the Injury Assessment Protocol sidebar. For more information on injury assessment, consult the reading list at the end of the book, which includes an excellent text that addresses how to evaluate musculoskeletal injury.

Role of Exercise

As an athletic trainer, you must do more than tape, brace, cast, or splint an injured patient; you have a responsibility to provide the patient with appropriate stretching and strengthening exercises. Preventing injury or eliminating its recurrence will be possible only when the patient has achieved normal strength, flexibility, and range of motion! We discuss in this book exercises that require minimal equipment. Have the rehabilitated patient who has met the criteria for returning to competition use them to maintain strength and flexibility.

Criteria for Returning to Competition

Although taping procedures facilitate a patient's return to physical activity, these adjunctive measures do not substitute for the patient's preinjury functional ability. After patients suffer an upper- or lower-extremity injury, they should regain strength, flexibility, and range of motion comparable to the uninjured side before continuing with the sport. If the injury involves the lower extremity, test the patient on functional activities that include running and cutting. For example, a patient displaying an **antalgic gait**, with or without tape, should not return to competition.

Criteria for Returning an Injured Patient to Competition

▶ The injured area has regained normal strength, flexibility, and range of motion when compared with the uninjured side.

▶ The patient performs functional tests, such as running, cutting, and other agility exercises, at full speed without limping.

▶ The patient's psychological condition demonstrates willingness and enthusiasm to return.

PREPARING FOR TAPING, CASTING, AND SPLINTING

Taping, casting, and splinting should occur in an environment that maximizes your effectiveness. Because you will devote many hours to this psychomotor task, you will optimize your clinical skills by preparing yourself, your facility, and your patients. Your preparation and the patient's cooperation are essential.

Casting and splinting should be performed in a temperature-controlled environment that has access to a sink with hot and cold running water, maximizes your efficiency, and allows for proper positioning of the patient. The amount of time it takes for fiberglass and plaster to harden is directly related to the ambient temperature of the room; the higher the temperature the less amount of time you have until the material hardens. As casting and splinting material hardens it becomes more difficult to work with, which is why it is extremely important to work in an environment that maximizes your efficiency. Proper positioning of the injured area while a splint or cast is being applied is vital to ensuring that the area heals in normal anatomical alignment.

Environment

Maintain the cleanliness and professional appearance of your taping, casting, and splinting area. It should have adequate illumination and ventilation. Because heat and humidity make it difficult to apply tape and fiberglass material, store your supplies in a cool environment.

Your work will require you to spend many hours performing psychomotor skills. Therefore, it is important to prepare a comfortable environment for when you are taping, casting, and splinting. Taping tables differ from treatment tables. In general, treatment tables are 72 inches (183 cm) long and 30 inches (76 cm) high; taping tables should be approximately 48 inches (122 cm) long and 35 inches (89 cm) high, depending on your height.

When traveling with a team, arrange an adequate facility for pregame taping. Taping from a bus seat or hotel bed can turn this pleasurable routine into an arduous and painful process.

Gender Considerations

Athletic training has attained the status of an allied health profession, and patients should be treated in a coeducational environment. In most practice settings you will care for both male and female patients. Applying protective taping, splinting, or casting to an opposite-gender patient rarely presents any difficulty, but you should always protect your patients' privacy. For example, the female patient should wear a halter top or sports bra during shoulder taping, and you can apply elastic wraps over tights to the hip and groin in both male and female patients.

Team travel away from home occasionally creates an inconvenience when preparing an area for pregame taping, and the difficulty sometimes increases when caring for opposite-gender patients. You have the option of waiting for patients to be properly clothed before entering the locker room to fulfill your taping responsibilities. Should time become a consideration, have the taping table removed from the locker room to an adjacent area. You can then tape your patients while the remainder of the team dresses for competition.

Preparation and Cooperation of the Patient

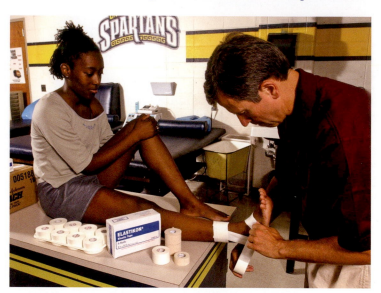

Figure 1.14 Attentive patient during ankle taping. Note how the patient sits with the ankle held at 90° of flexion.

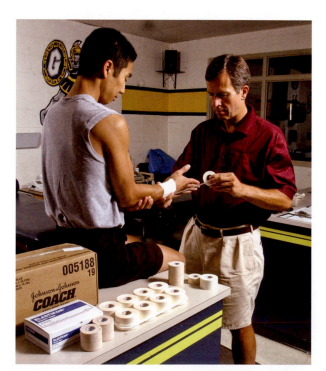

Figure 1.15 Attentive patient during wrist taping. Note how the patient stabilizes the forearm while the athletic trainer applies tape to the wrist.

Patients should sit or stand and pay attention when you tape the injured area (figures 1.14 and 1.15). An inattentive patient who is slouching or reclining on the taping table will fail to maintain the injured body part in an appropriate anatomical position. A sagging ankle or limp wrist will quickly cause you frustration and compromise the effectiveness of your procedure.

Before applying tape, make certain that the area is clean and, ideally, free of hair. Keep a barber's clipper handy in your taping area.

You may use an additional adherent when applying tape—many are available commercially—but it is not necessary if the body part is clean, shaved, and dry. When tape contacts bony prominences and muscle tendons, the resulting friction often produces blisters. To maximize the patient's comfort, apply friction pads with lubricant to these areas before using tape (figure 1.16). Pretaping underwrap may also prevent blistering, but it often causes the tape to slip (figure 1.17). For this reason, we recommend a minimal amount of underwrap, applied in conjunction with tape adherent.

APPLYING AND REMOVING TAPE

Here are several basic skills you must learn when applying and removing tape:

• *Tearing tape*: Although a seemingly simple task, tearing tape will present your first challenge. Developing this skill is often frustrating, particularly when your instructor prohibits you from using your teeth! To tear tape successfully, place your fingers close together at the site of the intended tear, pull the tape apart, and quickly snap your fingers in opposite directions (figure 1.18). If the tape becomes crimped or folded, its tensile strength increases exponentially, and it will be impossible to tear. If this occurs, move to a different point along the edge of the tape and try again.

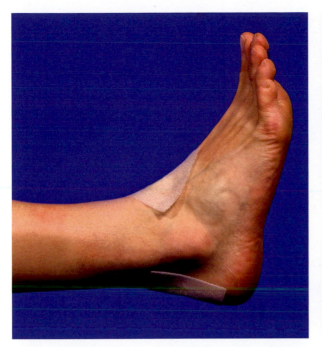

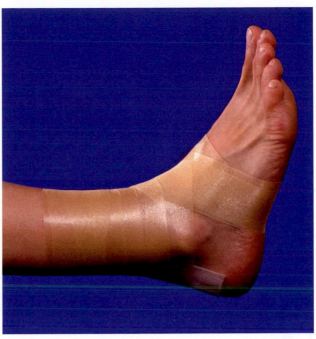

Figure 1.16   Friction pads placed over bony prominences or areas prone to irritation from tape. Place these pads over the tendons in the front and back of the ankle before taping to prevent cuts and abrasions.

Figure 1.17   Underwrap before tape application. For optimal adherence, apply the tape directly to the skin. For some patients, however, underwrap can prevent irritation or rashes that may result from the prolonged contact of tape with skin.

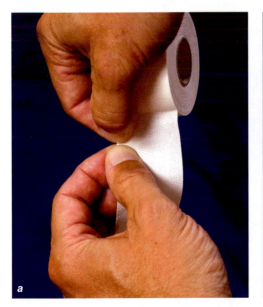

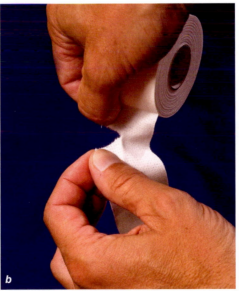

Figure 1.18   Technique for tearing nonelastic tape. *(a)* Place the fingers close together and follow with a quick, snapping motion in opposite directions. *(b)* The tape should tear, but if it becomes folded or crimped, move your fingers away from the folded area and try again. You can tear some elastic tape with the fingers, but you will need to cut other types with scissors.

- *Applying tape*: Begin taping by first supplying anchors that will secure the subsequent strips (figure 1.19). As you apply the tape, overlap the previous strip by one-half the width of the tape (figure 1.20). Whenever possible, tape from the **distal** to the **proximal** points of an extremity, using single strips. Avoid continuously unwinding the tape around an extremity because this technique may produce wrinkles and compromise circulation.

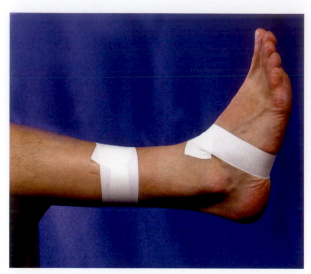

Figure 1.19 Application of anchor strips to start most taping procedures, illustrating anchor strips on the ankle before taping. Note the potential for irritation over the ankle tendons because of the absence of friction pads.

• *Removing tape:* Athletic trainers should be sure to remove all tape at the conclusion of practices or games. Use surgical scissors or commercially available tape cutters to cut the tape in an area with the least amount of bony prominence and greatest tissue compliance (figure 1.21). Pull back the tape with a slow, gentle motion while the skin is compressed (figure 1.22). Tape-removing agents are available

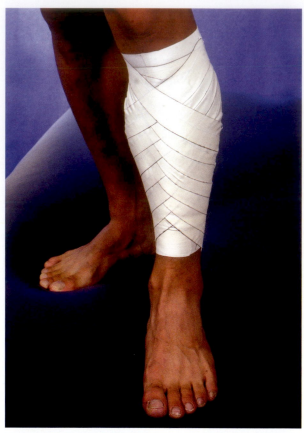

Figure 1.20 Overlapping strips of tape applied to the leg. Note how each strip overlaps the preceding strip by one-half the width of the tape. Tear each strip after application rather than apply the tape in a continuous fashion. Continuously applying nonelastic tape usually produces wrinkles and can constrict blood flow and normal muscle function. Normally, you may apply elastic tape and elastic wraps in a continuous manner.

to ease the process. You should monitor the skin for cuts, blisters, or signs of allergic reaction. Properly clean and dress cuts and blisters. If the patient develops a rash, you will need to find an alternative to treating the injury with tape.

We've included this general competency checklist to help instructors and students alike evaluate the knowledge, skills, and techniques necessary for effective injury assessment and taping.

Taping Competency Checklist

1. Determines mechanism of injury ☐
2. Ensures a clean, shaved body part ☐
3. Selects appropriate tape or wrap ☐
4. Properly positions patient and body part ☐
5. Correctly applies appropriate taping procedure ☐
6. Correctly instructs patient on tape removal ☐
7. Ensures the patient's compliance with appropriate exercise regimen ☐

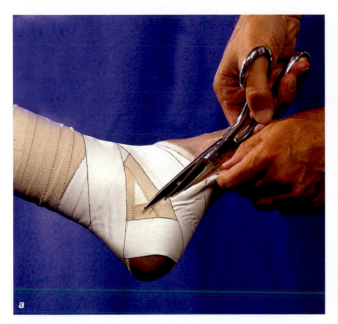

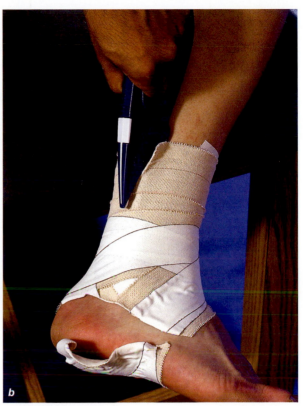

Figure 1.21 *(a)* Use surgical scissors with a blunt tip or a tape cutter to remove tape. *(b)* Cut the tape where it tends to be loose because of the anatomical configuration of the body part.

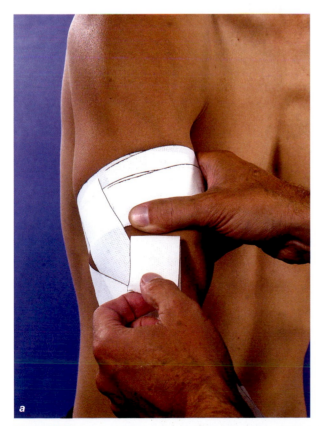

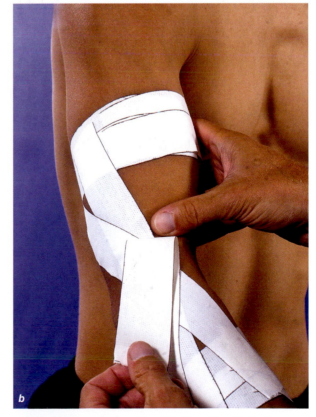

Figure 1.22 Appropriate removal of tape from skin. *(a)* Note how one hand supports the skin while the other *(b)* slowly removes the tape by pulling in a direction exactly opposite the stabilized skin.

APPLYING AND REMOVING CASTS AND SPLINTS

This section details the fundamental steps and important considerations that pertain to applying and removing fiberglass casts and splints.

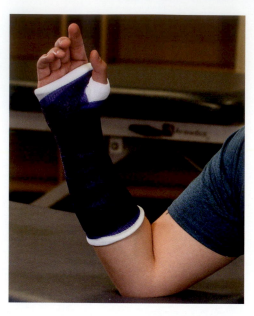

Application of a Fiberglass Cast

1. Based upon history, physical exam, and imaging studies, determine what type of cast should be applied.

2. Inspect the involved extremity and document the presence or absence of skin lesions, open wounds, and swelling.

   a. Presence of an open wound in an area that will be covered by the cast is a contraindication to applying the cast.

   b. If post-traumatic swelling is still present and the injury occurred less than 48 hours ago, it is contraindicated to apply a cast. If the injury occurred more than 48 hours ago, swelling is gradually decreasing, and the patient is capable of elevating the involved extremity, a cast can be applied. Manifestations of compartment syndrome must be reviewed.

3. Check and document distal neurovascular status for the involved and uninvolved extremity.

4. Cover the patient's clothing with a protective barrier.

5. To determine the amount of stockinette needed, measure about 4 inches (10 cm) beyond each end of the area that will be casted.

6. Apply stockinette and place each joint that will be immobilized in a functional position. Specific positions are as follows:

   a. Elbow: 90° of flexion (see figure 6.13a)

   b. Wrist: 30° of extension (see figure 7.22a)

   c. Thumb: midway between maximal radial and palmar abduction (see figure 7.22a)

   d. Hand: metacarpophalangeal joints in 70° of flexion and interphalangeal joints in full extension (see figure 7.19a)

   e. Knee: 15° to 30° of flexion

   f. Ankle: 0° of dorsiflexion (see figure 2.33a)

7. Smooth out any wrinkles in the stockinette. If needed, trim the stockinette over flexor surfaces.

8. Apply cast padding by beginning about 1 inch (2-3 cm) beyond the distal end of the area that will be casted. Roll the cast padding circumferentially from distal to proximal, making sure to overlap the previous layer by 50%. This will provide two layers of padding. Ideally you should have two to three layers of padding. The cast padding should extend about 1 inch (2-3 cm) beyond the proximal end of the area that will be casted (see figure 2.33e).

   a. Extra padding can be applied to protect bony prominences (e.g., ulnar styloid, olecranon process, medial malleoli, and lateral malleoli).

   b. Place extra padding at the proximal and distal edges of the area that will be casted.

     c. Too much padding on the flexor surface of a joint will increase the risk of skin irritation and skin breakdown.

     d. Excessive padding can compromise the ability of the cast to immobilize the injured area.

9. Apply fiberglass casting material by beginning about 1 inch (2-3 cm) in from the distal end of the cast padding. The fiberglass material should be rolled circumferentially from distal to proximal, overlapping the previous layer by 50%. Maintaining a small amount of uniform tension will reduce the risk of skin irritation, neurological injury, and vascular compromise (see figure 2.33*h*).

10. After applying two to three layers of fiberglass, confirm that functional positioning of the joints has been maintained. Using the palm and heel of the hand, mold the casting material as needed. Never use the fingertips when molding because they may create focal pressure points that increase the risk of skin irritation and pressure sores.

11. Prior to applying the final layer of fiberglass, fold the stockinette back over the previously applied fiberglass. The final layer of fiberglass should be applied in a distal to proximal direction. If necessary, mold the final layers of casting material.

12. Following cast application. recheck and document distal neurovascular status for the involved and uninvolved extremity.

 Video 1.1 demonstrates the preparation and application of a fiberglass cast.

Application of a Fiberglass Splint

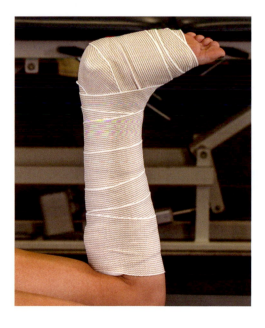

1. Based upon history, physical exam, and imaging studies, determine what type of splint should be applied.

2. Inspect the involved extremity and document the presence or absence of skin lesions, open wounds, and swelling.

3. Check and document distal neurovascular status for the involved and uninvolved extremity.

4. Cover the patient's clothing with a protective barrier.

5. To determine the amount of stockinette needed, measure about 4 inches (10 cm) beyond each end of the area that will be splinted.

6. Apply stockinette and place each joint that will be immobilized in a functional position. Specific positions are as follows:

     a. Elbow: 90° of flexion (see figure 6.13*a*)

     b. Wrist: 30° of extension (see figure 7.22*a*)

     c. Thumb: midway between maximal radial and palmar abduction (see figure 7.22*a*)

     d. Hand: metacarpophalangeal joints in 70° of flexion and interphalangeal joints in full extension (see figure 7.19*a*)

     e. Knee: 15° to 30° of flexion

     f. Ankle: 0° of dorsiflexion (see figure 2.32*a*)

7. Smooth out any wrinkles in the stockinette. If needed, trim the stockinette over flexor surfaces.

8. Apply cast padding by beginning about 1 inch (2-3 cm) beyond the distal end of the area that will be splinted. Roll the cast padding circumferentially from distal to proximal, making sure to overlap the previous layer by 50%. This will provide two layers of padding. Ideally you should have two to three layers of padding. The cast padding should extend about 1 inch (2-3 cm) beyond the proximal end of the area that will be splinted (see figure 2.32*d*).

   a. Extra padding can be applied to protect bony prominences (e.g., ulnar styloid, olecranon process, medial malleoli, and lateral malleoli).

   b. Place extra padding at the proximal and distal edges of the area that will be casted.

   c. Too much padding on the flexor surface of a joint will increase the risk of skin irritation and skin breakdown.

   d. Excessive padding can compromise the ability of the cast to immobilize the injured area.

9. The uninvolved extremity can be used to measure the length of the area that is being splinted. Add 1 to 2 inches (2.5-5 cm) to your measurement to accommodate for shrinkage of the cast that occurs due to molding and drying.

10. Prepare the fiberglass splint by unrolling the fiberglass to the desired length; this will create the first layer of the splint. The next layer is created by folding back the fiberglass material. Repeat this process until the splint is the desired thickness. The size of the patient, involved extremity, and desired strength of the splint determines the thickness. Guidelines for an average adult follow:

    a. Upper extremity splints should have 6 to 10 layers.

    b. Lower extremity splints should have 12 to 15 layers.

    c. Be advised that while adding layers will increase the strength of the splint, the splint will become bulkier and weigh more, and the risk of thermal injury increases.

11. Submerge the entire splint in room-temperature water. Keep the splint under water until the bubbling stops. Remove the splint, quickly squeeze out any excess water, and place the splint on the nonabsorbent blue side of the disposable underpad, which has been placed on a hard surface. Smooth out the splint to ensure that there are no wrinkles or air pockets.

12. Place the splint over the cast padding and, using the palm and heel of the hand, mold the splint to the extremity. Never use the fingertips when molding because they may create focal pressure points that increase the risk of skin irritation and pressure sores. While molding the splint, take care to ensure that functional positioning of the joint is been maintained (see figure 2.32*d*).

13. Fold the stockinette and cast padding back over the fiberglass splint. Secure the splint in place with an elastic wrap that is started at the distal end and rolled proximally. Overlapping the previous layer by 50% will provide uniform compression and ensure that the splint stays in the proper position. Overlapping the elastic wrap >50% will create focal areas of compression that increase the risk of skin irritation, neurological injury, vascular compromise, or thermal injury. Overlapping the elastic wrap <50% compromises the stability of the splint.

14. Following splint application, recheck and document distal neurovascular status for the involved and uninvolved extremity.

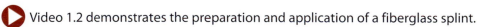 Video 1.2 demonstrates the preparation and application of a fiberglass splint.

Cast removal is best accomplished with use of a cast saw (see figure 1.23*a*) because it has an oscillating blade that is specially designed to cut hardened fiberglass and plaster. While the oscillating blade can damage the underlying soft tissue, the risk of injury is significantly less in comparison to that of a rotating saw blade. As the oscillating blade cuts the hard cast material, a significant amount of heat is generated, which has the

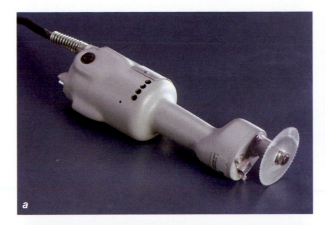

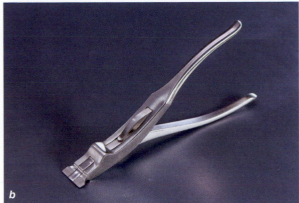

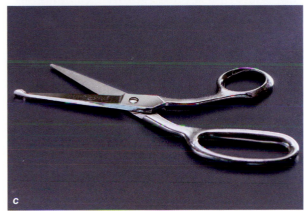

Figure 1.23 *(a)* Cast saw, *(b)* cast spreader, and *(c)* bandage scissors that are necessary for cast removal.

potential to burn the patient. Inserting a plastic cutting guard between the stockinette and skin and using proper cutting technique reduces the risk of soft-tissue injury. When cutting the fiberglass it is best to use the "up, over, and down" technique described here:

1. While holding the saw blade perpendicular to the cast (see figure 1.24*a*), apply gentle downward pressure until there is a sudden decrease in resistance, which indicates that the saw blade has cut through the cast.

2. Lift upwards to remove the saw blade. Once the saw blade is clear of the cast, move it over to the adjacent portion of the cast.

3. Once again, apply gentle downward pressure until the blade cuts through the cast.

4. Repeat this technique along the entire length of the cast.

5. Resist the temptation to "drag" or "push" the saw blade along the length of the cast because doing so significantly increases the risk of soft-tissue injury.

Cast removal is accomplished by making a longitudinal cut along the entire length of the cast followed by a similar cut on the opposing side of the cast. Once both cuts have been completed, a cast spreader (see figures 1.23*b* and 1.24*b*) can be used to separate the opposing halves of the cast, making it much easier to use bandage scissors (see figures 1.23*c* and 1.24*c*) to cut along the length of the underlying cast padding and stockinette.

 Video 1.3 demonstrates cast removal.

Splint removal is accomplished by first removing the elastic wrap that secures the splint in place. Next, the rigid splint is removed. When doing so it is extremely important to support the injured extremity to minimize any type of movement or stress that could compromise the healing that has taken place. Bandage scissors are used to cut along the entire length of the cast padding and stockinette, which is then removed.

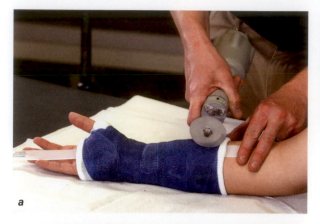

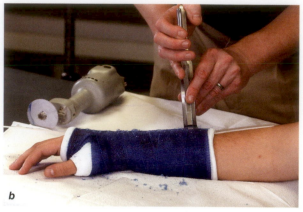

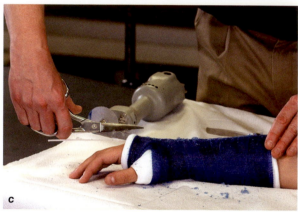

Figure 1.24 *(a)* Hold the cast saw blade perpendicular to the cast. *(b)* Cast spreader is used to separate the opposing edges of the cast. *(c)* Bandage scissors are used to cut the underlying cast padding and stockinette.

We've included the general competency checklist below to help instructors and students alike evaluate the knowledge, skills, and techniques necessary for effective injury assessment and casting or splinting.

The principles we have presented in this chapter will prepare you for the specific treatments that we discuss in the remaining chapters. Good luck as you begin your training in these gratifying psychomotor skills!

Casting and Splinting Competency Checklist

1. Determines mechanism of injury ☐
2. Ensures a clean body part that is free from open wounds ☐
3. Checks distal neurovascular status ☐
4. Selects appropriate splint or cast ☐
5. Properly positions patient and body part ☐
6. Correctly applies appropriate splinting or casting or combination procedure ☐
7. Checks distal neurovascular status ☐
8. Educates patient on signs and symptoms that would warrant removal of the splint or cast ☐
9. Correctly instructs patient on how to remove splint or how to seek assistance with removing a cast ☐

 Visit the web resource for checklists and video clips related to topics discussed in this chapter.

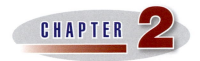

CHAPTER 2

The Foot, Ankle, and Leg

The foot contains a complex collection of bones, ligaments, and muscles. The 26 bones of the foot create several important joints. The talus and calcaneus form the subtalar joint, and the joining of the calcaneus with the cuboid and the talus with the navicular creates the midtarsal joint. The base of the five metatarsal bones and the tarsal bones form the tarsometatarsal (TMT) joints, while the heads of the metatarsals and the phalanges form the metatarsophalangeal (MP) joints. Each of the

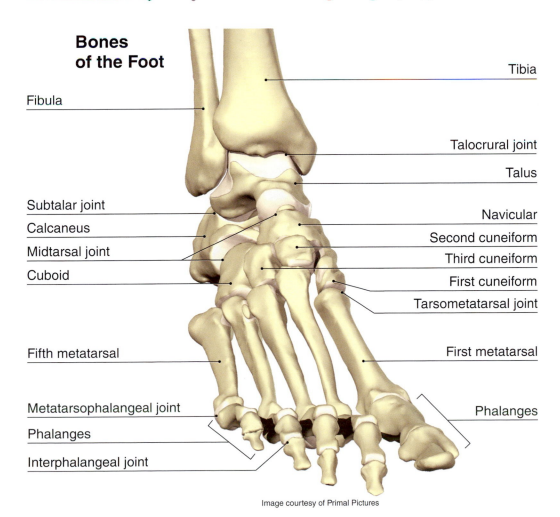

Bones of the Foot

Fibula

Subtalar joint

Calcaneus

Midtarsal joint

Cuboid

Fifth metatarsal

Metatarsophalangeal joint

Phalanges

Interphalangeal joint

Tibia

Talocrural joint

Talus

Navicular

Second cuneiform

Third cuneiform

First cuneiform

Tarsometatarsal joint

First metatarsal

Phalanges

Image courtesy of Primal Pictures

toes contains interphalangeal joints—one interphalangeal joint in the great toe and a proximal (PIP) and distal (DIP) interphalangeal joint in the remaining four toes. A multitude of small ligaments supports the joints in the foot.

The bones of the foot also create two arches. The first, a longitudinal arch, appears along the **medial** border of the foot. Patients with a pronounced (high) longitudinal arch are **pes cavus**, whereas those with flat feet have a **pes planus** foot. The second arch, formed by the heads of the five metatarsal bones, is the transverse arch.

The foot contains four muscle layers, known collectively as **intrinsic muscles**. The most **superficial** layer, the plantar fascia, maintains the longitudinal arch of the foot. The medial and **lateral** plantar nerves **innervate** the intrinsic muscles. These nerves continue into the toes between the metatarsal heads as **interdigital** nerves and are a common point of irritation in patients.

The **articulation** of the distal tibia and fibula with the talus, known as the talocrural joint, forms the ankle. The ankle and foot move by using a combination of the talocrural, subtalar, and midtarsal joints. Ankle **dorsiflexion** and **plantar flexion** occur primarily at the talocrural joint; **inversion** and **eversion** take place at the subtalar joint (figure 2.1). Foot **abduction** and **adduction** occur at the midtarsal joint. A combination (while non–weight-bearing) of ankle dorsiflexion, eversion, and foot abduction causes **pronation;** plantar flexion, inversion, and adduction result in **supination**.

Several ligaments reinforce the ankle. On the lateral side, the **anterior** talofibular, calcaneofibular, and posterior talofibular ligaments prevent excessive inversion. The broad and expansive deltoid ligament—a combination of four ligaments—provides stability to the medial aspect of the ankle and checks excessive eversion.

Extrinsic muscles acting on the toes and ankle have their **origin** in the leg. The anterior muscles—the tibialis anterior, extensor hallucis longus, extensor digitorum longus, and peroneus tertius—produce dorsiflexion and toe extension. The lateral muscles, consisting of the peroneus longus and peroneus brevis, cause eversion. The deep posterior-medial muscles, which include the tibialis posterior, flexor hallucis longus, and flexor digitorum longus, produce inversion and toe flexion. Plantar flexion occurs from the gastrocnemius, soleus, and plantaris muscles, also known as true **posterior** muscles. The gastrocnemius and soleus join with the calcaneus to form the Achilles tendon. The gastrocnemius and plantaris begin above the knee, but the

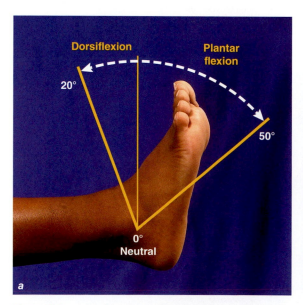
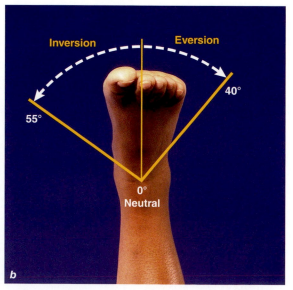

Figure 2.1   (a) Ankle plantar flexion and dorsiflexion ranges of motion; (b) ankle inversion and eversion ranges of motion.

soleus originates in the leg. This distinction will be significant during the discussion of stretching exercises for the ankle.

The ankle contains several **retinacula** that hold the tendons of the extrinsic muscles to the leg as they cross the ankle and pass into the foot. The extensor retinacula will be relevant when you use tape to alleviate the discomfort of shin splints.

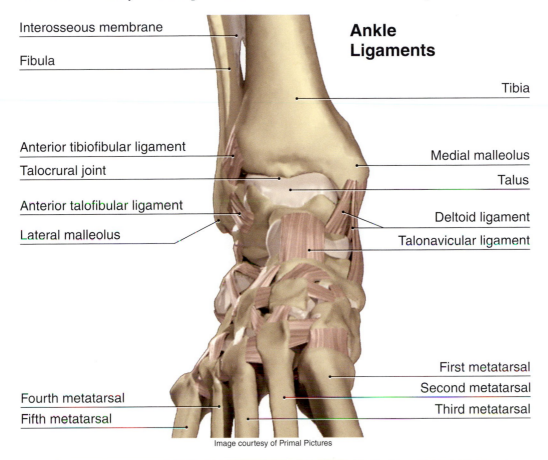

Interosseous membrane

Fibula

Ankle Ligaments

Tibia

Anterior tibiofibular ligament

Talocrural joint

Anterior talofibular ligament

Lateral malleolus

Medial malleolus

Talus

Deltoid ligament

Talonavicular ligament

Fourth metatarsal

Fifth metatarsal

First metatarsal

Second metatarsal

Third metatarsal

Image courtesy of Primal Pictures

Key Foot, Ankle, and Leg Palpation Landmarks

Lateral Aspect
- Anterior talofibular ligament
- Calcaneofibular ligament
- Posterior talofibular ligament
- Fifth metatarsal
- Lateral malleolus

Medial Aspect
- Deltoid ligament
- Longitudinal arch
- Medial malleolus

Anterior Aspect
- Anterior tibiofibular ligament

Posterior Aspect
- Achilles tendon
- Gastrocnemius muscle
- Soleus muscle

Plantar Surface
- Plantar fascia
- Transverse arch
- Calcaneus
- Sesamoid bone

Dorsal Surface
- First metatarsophalangeal joint

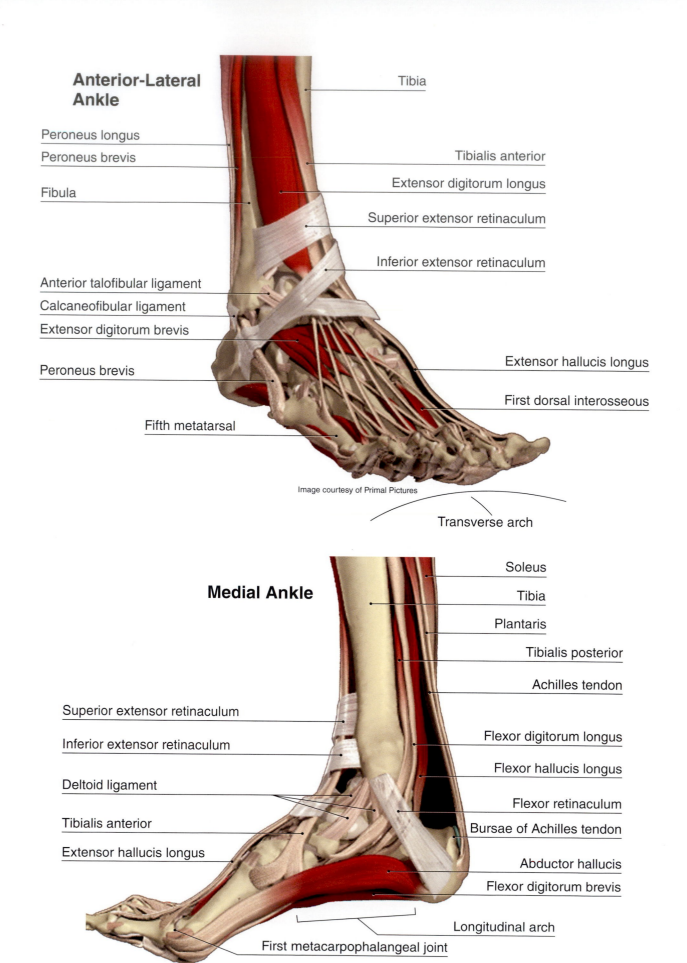

Anterior-Lateral Ankle

Peroneus longus

Peroneus brevis

Fibula

Anterior talofibular ligament

Calcaneofibular ligament

Extensor digitorum brevis

Peroneus brevis

Fifth metatarsal

Tibia

Tibialis anterior

Extensor digitorum longus

Superior extensor retinaculum

Inferior extensor retinaculum

Extensor hallucis longus

First dorsal interosseous

Image courtesy of Primal Pictures

Transverse arch

Medial Ankle

Superior extensor retinaculum

Inferior extensor retinaculum

Deltoid ligament

Tibialis anterior

Extensor hallucis longus

Soleus

Tibia

Plantaris

Tibialis posterior

Achilles tendon

Flexor digitorum longus

Flexor hallucis longus

Flexor retinaculum

Bursae of Achilles tendon

Abductor hallucis

Flexor digitorum brevis

Longitudinal arch

First metacarpophalangeal joint

Image courtesy of Primal Pictures

Posterior Muscles

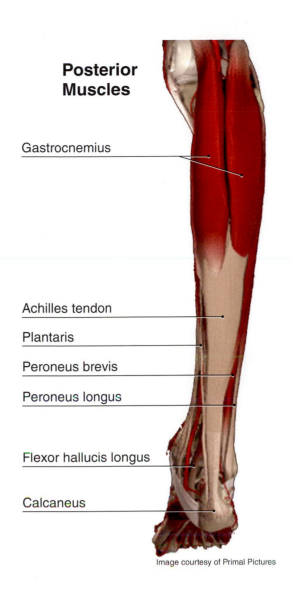

Gastrocnemius

Achilles tendon

Plantaris

Peroneus brevis

Peroneus longus

Flexor hallucis longus

Calcaneus

Image courtesy of Primal Pictures

Surface Anatomy

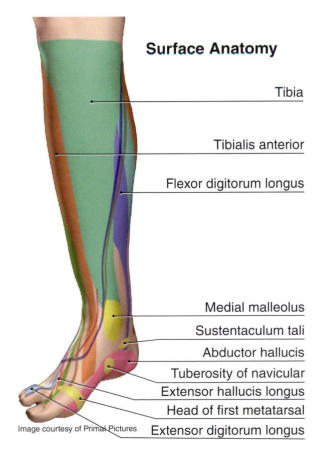

Tibia

Tibialis anterior

Flexor digitorum longus

Medial malleolus

Sustentaculum tali

Abductor hallucis

Tuberosity of navicular

Extensor hallucis longus

Head of first metatarsal

Extensor digitorum longus

Image courtesy of Primal Pictures

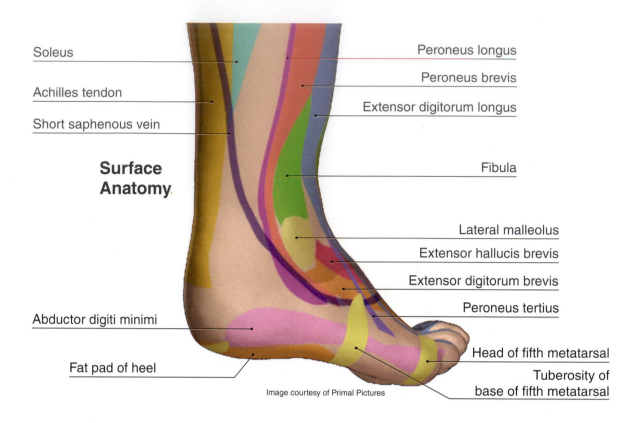

Surface Anatomy

Soleus

Achilles tendon

Short saphenous vein

Abductor digiti minimi

Fat pad of heel

Peroneus longus

Peroneus brevis

Extensor digitorum longus

Fibula

Lateral malleolus

Extensor hallucis brevis

Extensor digitorum brevis

Peroneus tertius

Head of fifth metatarsal

Tuberosity of base of fifth metatarsal

Image courtesy of Primal Pictures

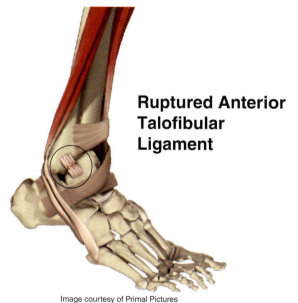

Ruptured Anterior Talofibular Ligament

Image courtesy of Primal Pictures

ANKLE SPRAINS

Physical activity places excessive stress on the foot and ankle and renders this region of the body highly susceptible to injury. Ankle sprains will be the most common injury that you encounter.

Ankle sprains result from excessive inversion or eversion. Inversion sprains are more common because of the bone and ligament configuration of the joint. The four ligaments of the deltoid complex are stronger than the three separate, laterally placed ligaments, and the mortise created by the fibula extends more distally than that of the tibia. These factors limit eversion and account for the higher incidence of inversion ankle sprains. A less common type of sprain is the "**high ankle sprain**," which involves injury to the anterior tibiofibular ligament and interosseous membrane. The mechanism of this injury is forced dorsiflexion and external rotation. You can support the sprained ankle by applying tape, braces, walking boots, or a combination of the three treatments.

▶ Video 2.1 demonstrates application of compression with an elastic wrap, an elastic wrap to secure an ice bag, and an elastic wrap with a horseshoe pad to reduce swelling.

Closed Basketweave Taping

Begin the closed basketweave procedure by applying anchor strips and follow with a succession of interlocking vertical and horizontal strips. Complete the taping with one or more heel-lock strips on the medial and lateral aspects of the ankle (figure 2.2). With an inversion sprain, start the vertical strips on the medial side of the leg and pull to the lateral aspect. For an eversion injury, begin the vertical strips on the lateral leg and pull to the medial side. Note that horizontal and vertical strips pertain to the anatomical position of the body (i.e., standing erect).

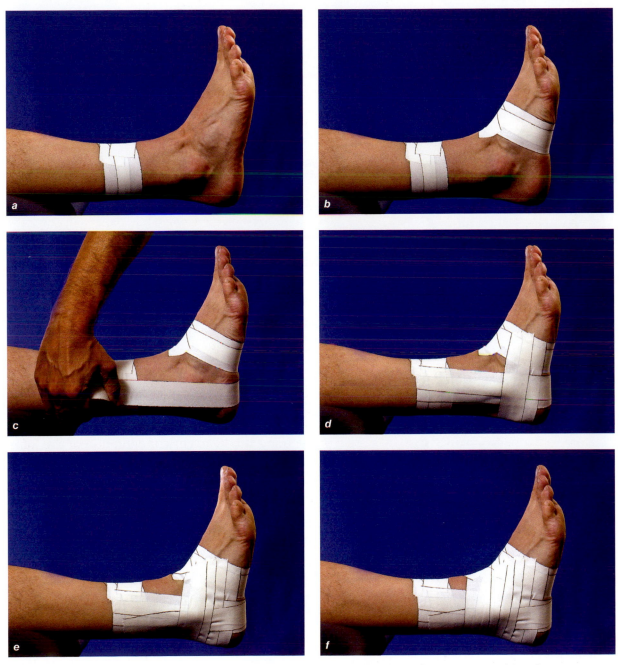

Figure 2.2   Closed basketweave taping procedure for the ankle. The patient holds the ankle in 90° of dorsiflexion. For ease of illustration, these photos do not show the use of friction pads. Place two anchor strips on *(a)* the distal leg and, possibly, *(b)* around the foot. Because the foot anchors frequently cause constriction and discomfort, consider them optional. To prevent or protect inversion sprains, *(c)* apply a stirrup strip from the medial aspect of the leg and pull under the heel to the lateral aspect of the leg. For eversion sprains, the direction of the stirrup would be the opposite, from lateral leg to medial leg. Place a horizontal horseshoe strip from the medial to lateral aspect of the foot and *(d)* follow by another stirrup in a weaving fashion. *(e-f)* Continue this process until you have applied three stirrups.   *(continued)*

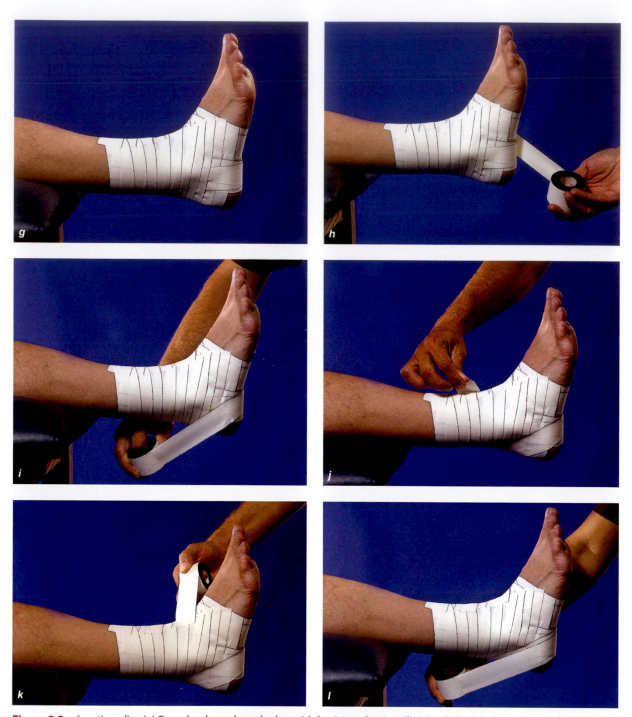

Figure 2.2 *(continued)*   *(g)* Completely enclose the leg with horizontal strips. *(h-j)* Apply heel locks to the medial and lateral aspects of the ankle one at a time (application to the lateral side of the ankle is shown here). Note how to apply the lateral heel lock by pulling in an upward direction. *(k-n)* A more advanced variation would incorporate heel locks in a figure-eight pattern. Note how to apply the lateral heel lock by pulling in an upward direction and the medial heel lock by pulling in a downward direction.   *(continued)*

▶ Video 2.2 demonstrates the closed basketweave taping procedure for the ankle.

Be aware that applying an anchor too tight around the foot is the most frequent error with this taping procedure. Because the foot spreads when supporting the weight of the body, a constricting distal anchor can be extremely uncomfortable for the patient. Apply this anchor as close to the ankle as possible. You can even omit it for patients requiring greater dexterity.

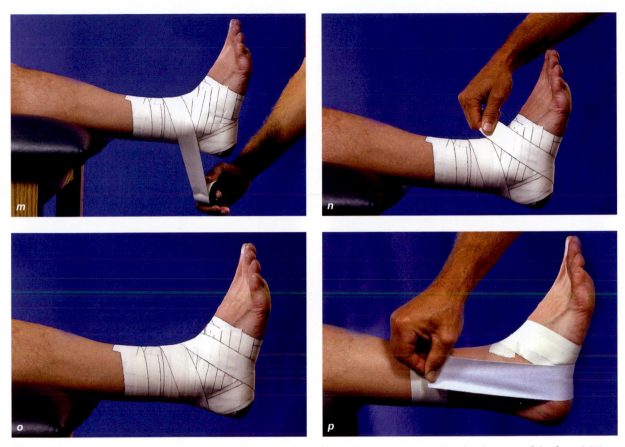

Figure 2.2 *(continued)* *(o)* The final product supports the ankle without constricting the distal aspect of the foot. *(p)* You can provide additional support with the application of a 2- or 3-inch (5.1 or 7.6 cm) moleskin stirrup before applying the closed basketweave.

Taping Variations and Alternatives

Purchase large rolls of cloth wrap that can be cut into lengths of 72 inches (about 180 cm). Combining the cloth wrap with a small amount of white tape will provide adequate support (figure 2.3). Cloth wraps do not work as well as nonelastic tape, but they are a reasonable, cost-effective alternative. For the athletic training student, cloth

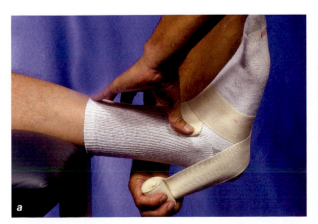
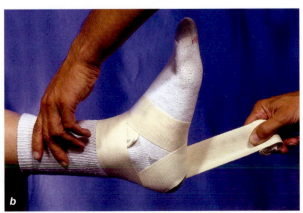

Figure 2.3 Apply a cloth ankle wrap as a less expensive (although less effective) alternative to closed basketweave taping. Apply this procedure over a sock with the ankle positioned in 90° of dorsiflexion. First, *(a-b)* use a figure-eight pattern with heel locks incorporated in an upward direction for the lateral aspect and a downward direction for the medial aspect. *(continued)*

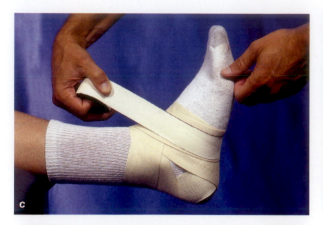

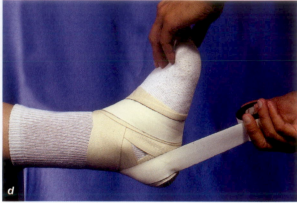

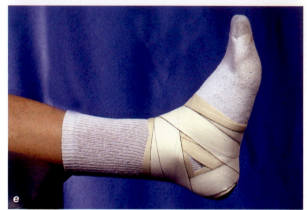

Figure 2.3   *(continued)*   *(c-e)* Trace with nonelastic tape.

wraps provide an excellent way to practice the complex figure-eight and heel-lock patterns without the expense or waste of adhesive tape. Cloth wraps can be applied alone or supplemented with nonelastic tape.

You can also use the closed basketweave procedure with a combination of mole-skin (figure 2.2) or nonelastic and elastic tape (figure 2.4). This alternative may be acceptable for patients who want some protection but do not require the additional support of an all-white taping procedure.

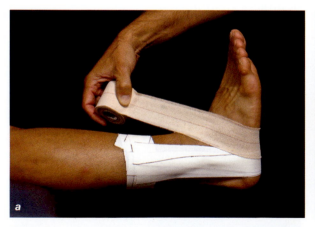

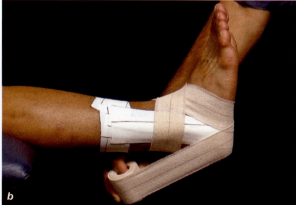

Figure 2.4   Nonelastic and elastic tape combination. For less support, *(a-b)* use stirrups of nonelastic tape and apply both a figure-eight pattern and heel locks with elastic tape.   *(continued)*

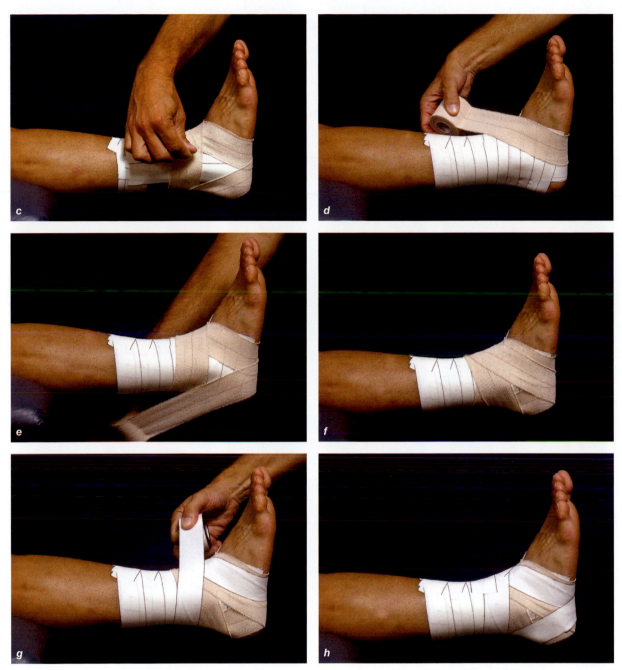

Figure 2.4 *(continued)* *(c)* Use elastic tape to encircle the leg completely to the anchor strips; you then have the option of repeating the figure eight and heel locks with nonelastic tape. *(d-f)* A variation that would provide additional support uses nonelastic tape for all stirrup and horseshoe strips and then includes elastic tape to apply the figure eight and heel locks. *(g-h)* Elastic tape could complete the procedure, or you could repeat the figure eight and heel locks with nonelastic tape.

Open Basketweave Taping

This taping technique supports and compresses the acutely injured ankle. Although similar to the closed basketweave, the open technique leaves the **dorsum** of the foot uncovered (figure 2.5). In some cases, you can cover the taping procedure with an elastic wrap to supply more compression. Instruct the patient to remove the elastic wrap at night but to leave the taping procedure in place.

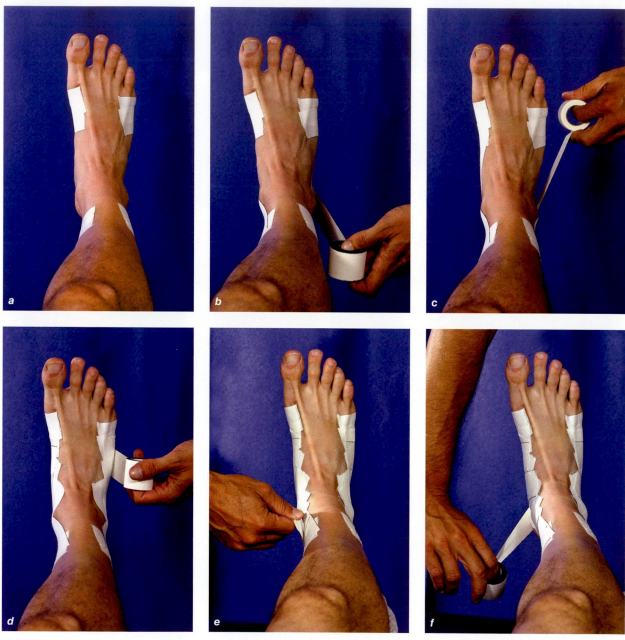

Figure 2.5   Open basketweave taping to compress and support an acutely injured ankle. *(a)* The procedure begins with proximal and distal anchors, but leave them open on the anterior leg and the dorsum of the foot. *(b)* For an inversion sprain, pull the stirrup strips from the medial to lateral aspects of the leg. *(c)* Apply the horseshoe strips in a manner similar to the closed basketweave, giving special attention to leaving the anterior leg and dorsum of the foot open. *(d-e)* Apply stirrups and horseshoe strips to enclose completely the plantar surface of the foot and the posterior aspect of the leg. Use single heel locks for *(f)* the medial and   *(continued)*

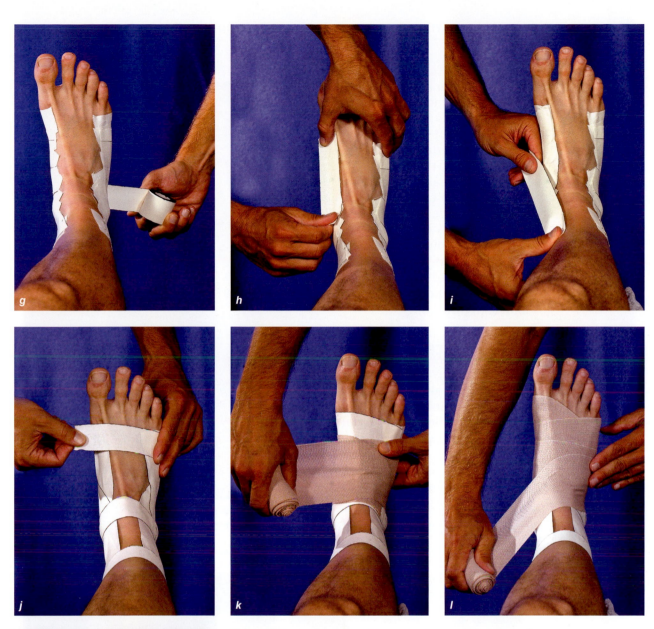

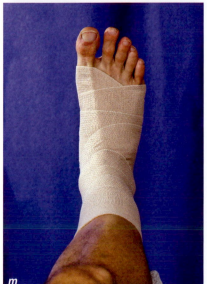

Figure 2.5 *(continued)* *(g)* lateral ankle. *(h-i)* Apply anchor strips to the anterior leg and dorsum of the foot. *(j)* Three horizontal strips secure the procedure, although you should instruct the patient to remove these strips if the ankle begins to ache from significant swelling. *(k-m)* Finally, apply an elastic wrap to secure the open basketweave and to offer additional compression to the acutely injured ankle. Remove the wrap when applying ice and when the patient sleeps.

 Video 2.3 demonstrates the open basketweave taping procedure for an acutely sprained ankle.

Because you apply the open basketweave taping procedure to support an acutely sprained ankle, you also may have to fit and provide the patient with crutches. The crutches should be fit so that they are 6 inches (15.2 cm) lateral and anterior to the feet and permit two to three finger widths of space between the axillae and the axillary pads of the crutches. The elbows should be flexed to about 20° to 30°, and you should instruct the patient to bear most of the weight with the hands, not in the axillae (figure 2.6).

Ankle Braces

Lace braces have become a popular substitute for ankle tape, especially when a clinician is unavailable (figure 2.7). These commercial supports can also supplement the taping procedure. The brace, normally applied over the sock, often uses lateral stays for reinforcement.

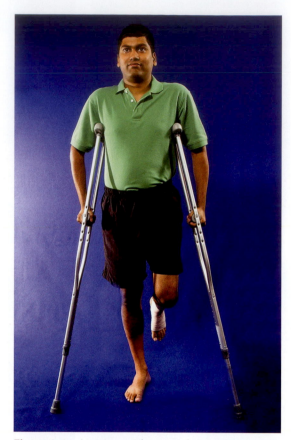

Figure 2.6   A patient with an antalgic gait should be fitted with crutches. The hands, not the axillae, should bear most of the weight.

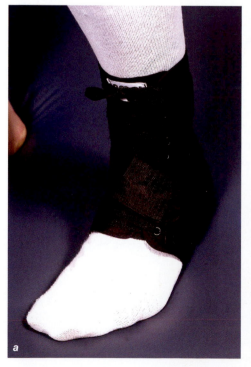

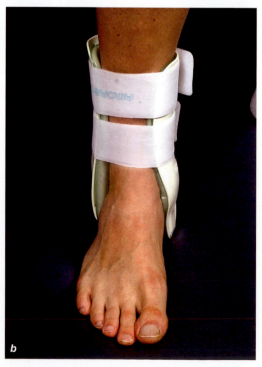

Figure 2.7   *(a-b)* Commercially available ankle braces that are alternatives to taping. The brace permits normal plantar flexion and dorsiflexion while limiting excessive inversion and eversion.

Walking Boot

Walking boots provide the opportunity to immobilize the ankle in an anatomical neutral position. The rigid nature of ankle boots affords more protection than ankle taping and bracing for the acutely injured ankle. The added support allows early weight bearing, which can offset detrimental effects such as atrophy of the muscles that result from not bearing weight. Walking boots are particularly useful in managing high ankle sprains through reduction in the load on the anterior tibiofibular ligament. Walking boots are available either as a nonadjustable version (figure 2.8) that maintains the ankle in a neutral position or an adjustable version (figure 2.9) that allows the clinician to manipulate the amount of range of motion permitted. Adjustable walking boots are beneficial in gradually increasing range of motion, which can assist with transitioning the patient from the walking boot to more normal gait patterns.

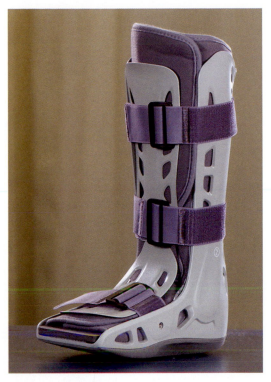

Figure 2.8 Commercially produced nonadjustable walking boot.

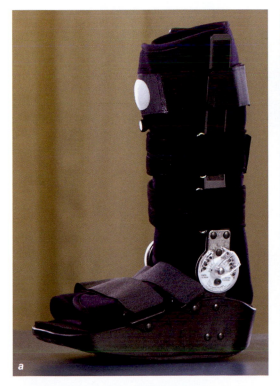

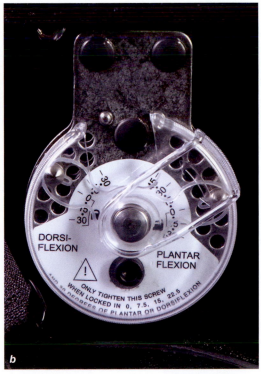

Figure 2.9 *(a)* Commercially produced adjustable walking boot and *(b)* close-up of adjustable range of motion dial on adjustable walking boot.

Ankle Exercises

Ankle exercises should restore or maintain normal flexibility, strength, and balance. A loss of normal ankle dorsiflexion often results from ankle sprains. Patients recovering from these injuries should stretch the ankle muscles and pay special attention to the gastrocnemius and soleus.

Figure 2.10 illustrates techniques for stretching the gastrocnemius and soleus muscles. Because the gastrocnemius begins on the femur, the patient first stretches with the knee completely extended. The patient continues by repeating the exercise with the knee flexed. The flexed knee shortens the gastrocnemius and isolates the soleus muscle, which originates from the tibia and fibula. Using a wedge board will also effectively stretch these muscles. The patient can manually stretch the remaining ankle muscles. Instruct your patients to perform **static stretching**—a stretch without movement for 10 to 15 seconds—for these and all exercises that we present in this book.

Strengthening exercises for the major muscle groups acting on the ankle implement elastic bands. The patient simply performs inversion, eversion, plantar flexion, and dorsiflexion against the resistance of the band (figure 2.11). The methods for strength-

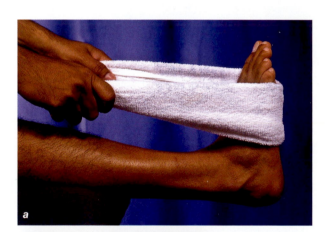

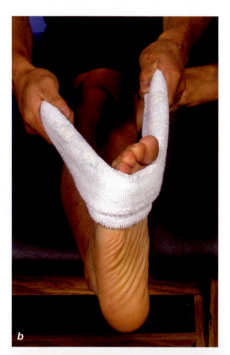

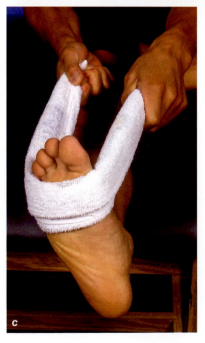

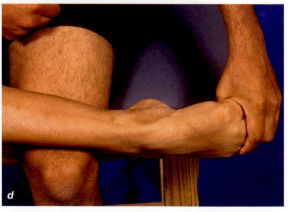

Figure 2.10 *(a)* Stretching the gastrocnemius leg muscle using a towel. The patient should dorsiflex the ankle with his or her own muscles and use the towel to provide an additional stretch. This stretch should also combine *(b)* ankle inversion and *(c)* eversion; repeat all three stretches with the knee flexed to 90° and with the leg hanging over the end of the table to isolate the soleus muscle. *(d)* Stretch the anterior ankle muscles by having the patient manually move the ankle into plantar flexion.

Figure 2.11 Ankle strengthening exercises with elastic material. Move the ankle into *(a)* inversion, *(b)* eversion, *(c)* plantar flexion, and *(d)* dorsiflexion against the resistance of the material. *(e)* Repeat plantar flexion with the knee flexed to 90° to isolate the soleus muscle.

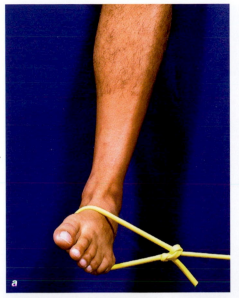
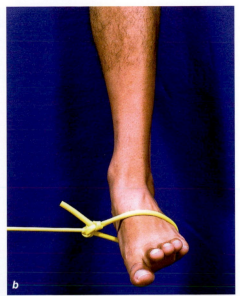

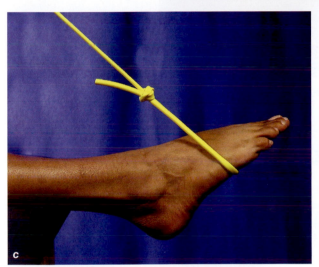
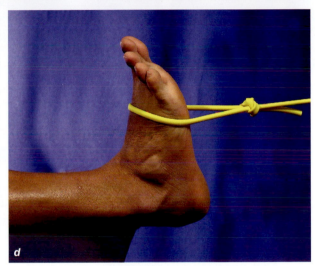

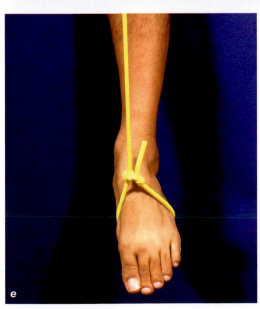

ening the ankle are similar to stretching exercises. The patient should execute plantar flexion with the knee both extended and flexed to isolate the gastrocnemius and soleus, respectively. We suggest that the patient complete three sets of at least 10 repetitions, with resistance adjusted to his or her tolerance, for all the strengthening exercises in this book. The reading list provides references to more sophisticated protocols for progressive resistance exercise.

An ankle injury will often compromise a patient's balance and proprioception. Balance devices are available to address these problems. You can also treat balance and proprioception deficits by having the patient stand on one leg with the eyes open and then closed (figure 2.12). Increase the difficulty of this exercise by applying light pressure to the shoulders from four random directions when the patient's eyes are shut.

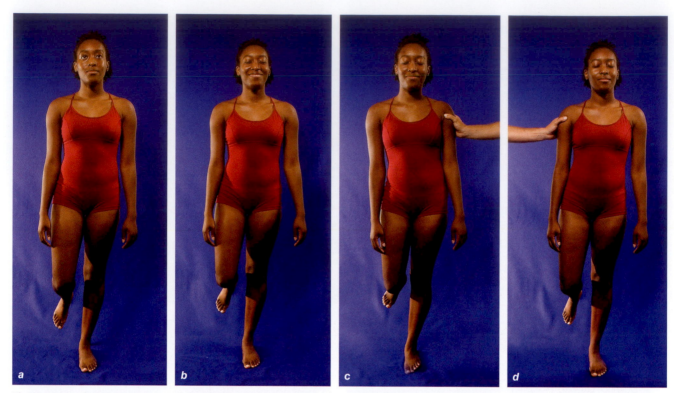

Figure 2.12 Proprioceptive exercises for the ankle. The patient begins by balancing on one leg with *(a)* the eyes open and then *(b)* closed. *(c-d)* Increase the difficulty by applying a light force from an unknown direction. The patient must contract the leg muscles to maintain balance.

ACHILLES TENDON STRAINS AND TENDINITIS

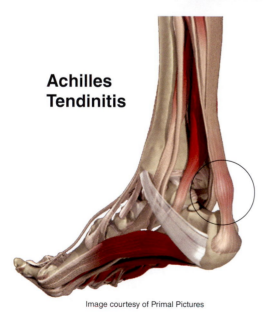

Achilles Tendinitis

Image courtesy of Primal Pictures

Running and jumping stress the Achilles tendon, the attachment of the gastrocnemius and soleus muscles to the heel. Achilles tendon **strains** and **tendinitis** are common athletic injuries. Older patients and those who are infrequently physically active occasionally rupture this tendon completely.

Acute overstretching or a forceful contraction of the gastrocnemius and soleus muscles causes an Achilles tendon strain. Tendinitis tends to be an **overuse injury** that often occurs when patients run or jump extensively. With either injury, the clinician should alleviate the patient's discomfort by applying tape to limit excessive dorsiflexion.

Achilles Tendon Rupture (Third-Degree Strain)

Ruptures of the Achilles tendon are most often seen in middle-aged males as a result of a direct trauma, forced dorsiflexion of the plantar flexed foot, or a strong push-off with knee extension and plantar flexion. This injury often occurs in sports such as basketball and sprint starts with explosive movements. A complete tear is noted in the majority of cases; however, partial tears can occur in some patients.

Treatment can be conservative with immobilization of the foot and ankle in a short leg cast with the ankle in a plantar flexed position for 8-12 weeks, as depicted in figure 2.13; however, this treatment method does have a higher rate of re-rupture compared to operative treatment. Some studies have suggested functional recovery is improved with early mobilization and rehabilitation.

Achilles Tendon Taping

Determine the amount of dorsiflexion that produces tendon discomfort. The patient should slightly plantar flex and maintain this position during the procedure. The taping consists of applying anchors around the leg and foot and a series of strips to limit dorsiflexion (see figure 2.14). Elastic tape is the best material because it will guarantee that dorsiflexion will not come to an abrupt end. You may also supplement the taping procedure by inserting a 1/4-inch (0.6-cm) heel lift in *both* shoes. When the patient uses heel lifts, be certain that he or she regularly performs stretching exercises to prevent adaptive shortening of the Achilles tendons.

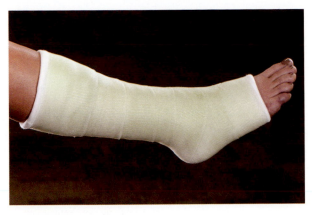

Figure 2.13   Short leg cast with the ankle in a plantar flexed position.

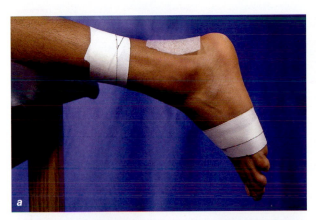

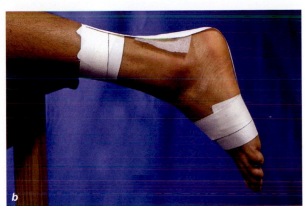

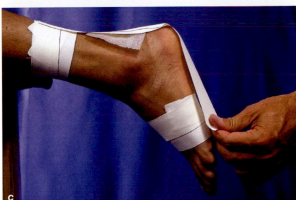

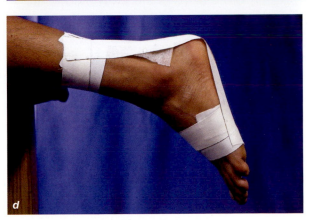

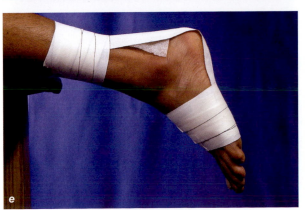

Figure 2.14   Taping procedure applied to limit extremes of dorsiflexion and, thus, to protect a strained or inflamed Achilles tendon. Identify the desired amount of dorsiflexion limitation and position the ankle accordingly. *(a)* Apply anchor strips proximally and distally with a friction pad to protect the Achilles tendon. *(b-d)* Supply three strips in an X fashion across the ankle to limit dorsiflexion. *(e)* Apply proximal and distal anchors.   *(continued)*

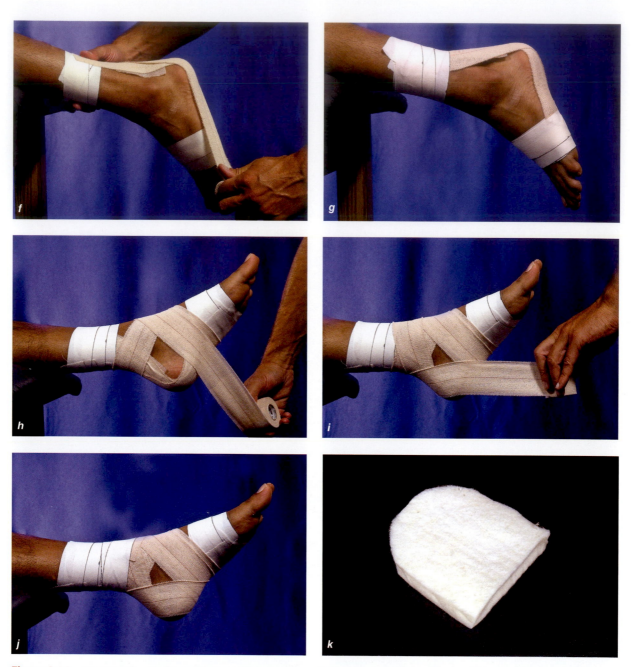

Figure 2.14 *(continued)* *(f-g)* Vary this procedure by using elastic tape to limit dorsiflexion. This would create a softer end point for limiting dorsiflexion. *(h-j)* Secure the entire procedure by applying both a figure eight and heel locks with elastic tape. *(k)* Supplement the procedure with a heel lift that can be placed in the patient's shoe. Place the lift in both shoes to avoid creating a leg length discrepancy.

▶ Video 2.4 demonstrates a taping procedure to limit dorsiflexion to support the strained Achilles tendon.

If full range of movement and agility is required of the foot and ankle (after, for example, a calf muscle strain)—and especially if the sport is played on an uneven surface—elastic kinesiology tape can be applied instead (figure 2.15).

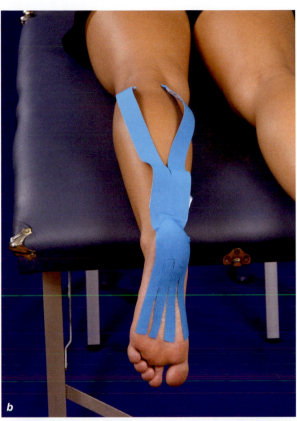

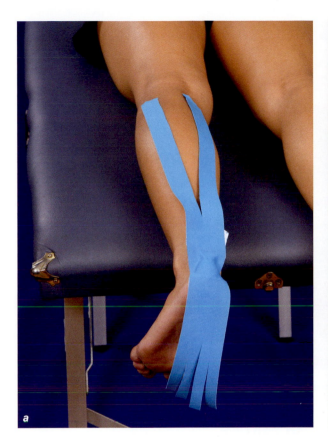

Figure 2.15 Kinesiology taping for gastrocnemius strains, Achilles tendonitis, or arch problems. *(a)* Start with the foot in dorsiflexion while the patient is prone with the foot off the table. Measure the tape from the distance of the top of the calf to the distal arch (metatarsal heads) and then cut. Cut four slit fans in arch section and a Y in the calf section. *(b)* Rip the backing from the tape, apply it at the heel, and stretch the tape to full tension across the arch to the base of the metatarsals. Rub the tape to activate adhesive. *(c)* Holding the heel piece securely, apply tape to medial and lateral gastrocnemius with minimal (15%-25%) stretch.

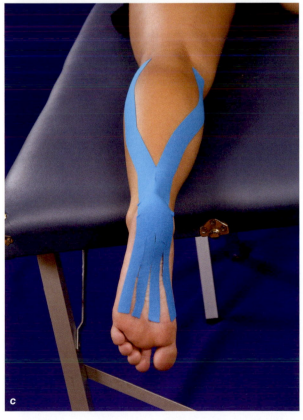

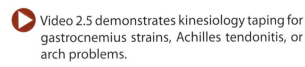 Video 2.5 demonstrates kinesiology taping for gastrocnemius strains, Achilles tendonitis, or arch problems.

Achilles Tendon Exercises

The exercises for the ankle are also appropriate for the Achilles tendon when the patient gives special attention to stretching and strengthening the gastrocnemius and soleus muscles (see figures 2.10 and 2.11).

ARCH STRAINS AND PLANTAR FASCIITIS

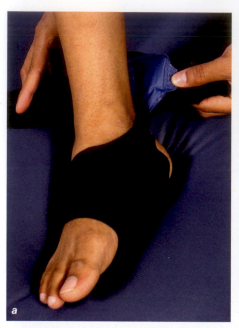
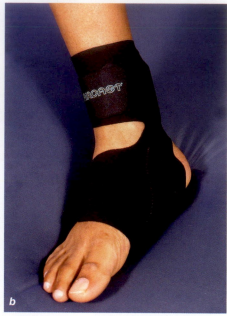

Physically active people with a pes cavus foot experience strains to the arch or plantar fascia. Excessive running or jumping causes an arch strain. In addition, running, and particularly the continual stress that it places on the foot, precipitates **plantar fasciitis**. Poorly constructed and improperly fitted athletic footwear can also cause these injuries. Some patients will experience relief from a commercially available plantar fasciitis brace (figure 2.16).

Figure 2.16   *(a-b)* A commercially produced brace that can help alleviate pain associated with plantar fasciitis.

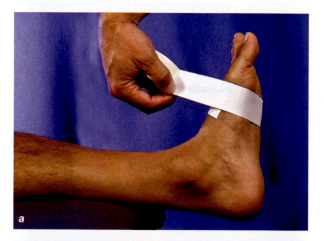

Arch Taping

Support the longitudinal arch with a simple taping procedure (figure 2.17) or a more complex X-arch taping procedure (figure 2.18). The simple procedure employs three or four strips placed circularly around the foot. To complete an X-arch taping, place an anchor strip around the metatarsal heads and successively overlap strips from the anchor, around the heel, and back to the anchor.

 Video 2.6 demonstrates the simple and x-arch taping procedures to support the longitudinal arch.

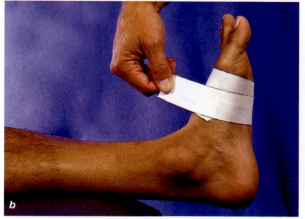
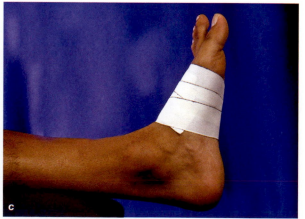

Figure 2.17   Simple taping to support the longitudinal arch. *(a-b)* Apply the tape by starting on the dorsum of the foot and then move in a lateral direction to lift, ultimately, the longitudinal arch. *(c)* Three or four strips will normally be adequate to support the longitudinal arch.

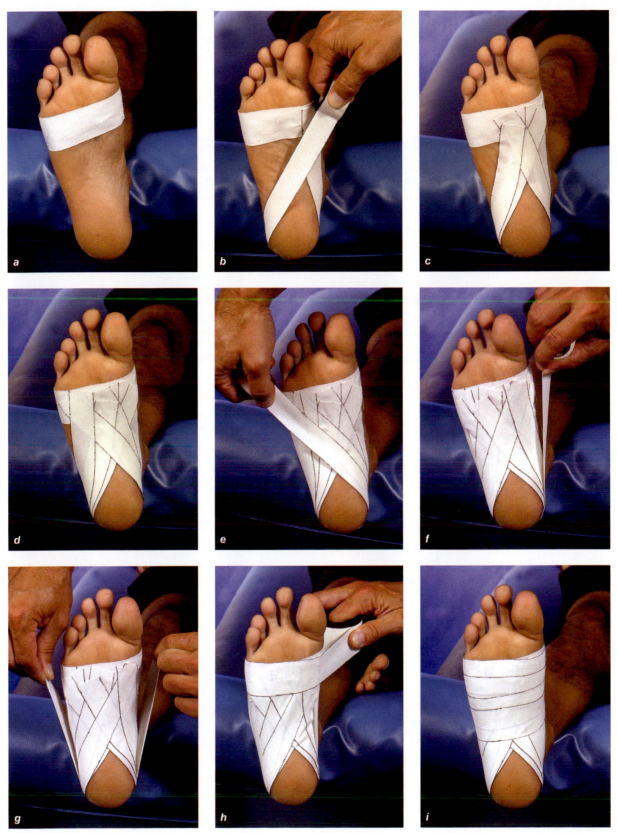

Figure 2.18 X-arch taping to support the longitudinal arch. *(a)* Following an anchor strip, *(b-c)* apply tape from the base of the great toe, around the heel, and back to the starting point. *(d)* Place subsequent strips from the medial to lateral aspect of the plantar surface of the foot. *(e-f)* Overlap strips from the lateral to medial aspect of the foot. *(g)* Apply a horseshoe strip from the lateral anchor to the medial anchor. *(h-i)* Complete the procedure with strips that mimic the simple arch taping procedure described in figure 2.17.

A longitudinal arch pad may make this taping more efficacious (figure 2.19).

For a more lasting application and rigid arch support, use strap taping instead (figure 2.20). Strap taping may last for a few days and does not have to be reapplied during sport. Strap taping of the arch also does not require an underwrap on the foot, and this is especially good for patients who wear tight or constricted shoes, patients who would normally use custom orthotics, or patients who perform barefooted.

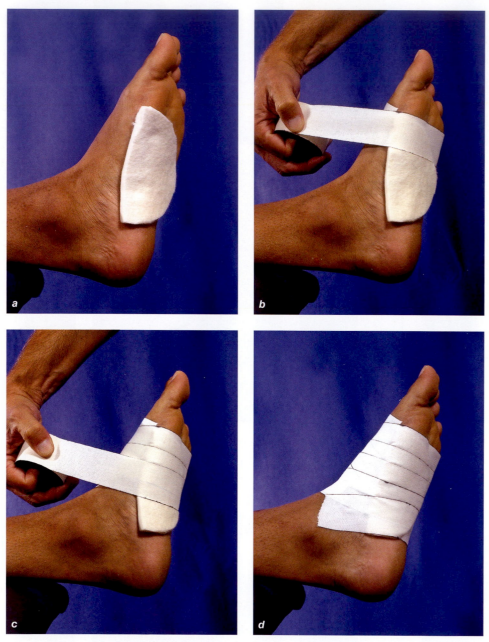

Figure 2.19   *(a)* Fashion a longitudinal arch pad from soft padding material and use it to support the patient with a high (pes cavus) longitudinal arch. *(b-d)* Secure the arch pad to the foot using the simple arch taping described in figure 2.17.

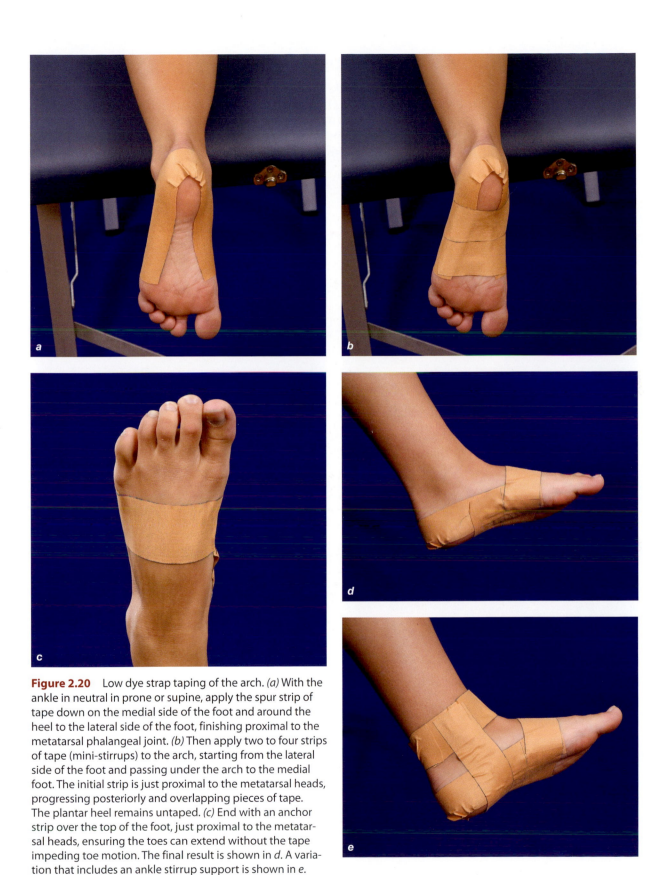

Figure 2.20 Low dye strap taping of the arch. *(a)* With the ankle in neutral in prone or supine, apply the spur strip of tape down on the medial side of the foot and around the heel to the lateral side of the foot, finishing proximal to the metatarsal phalangeal joint. *(b)* Then apply two to four strips of tape (mini-stirrups) to the arch, starting from the lateral side of the foot and passing under the arch to the medial foot. The initial strip is just proximal to the metatarsal heads, progressing posteriorly and overlapping pieces of tape. The plantar heel remains untaped. *(c)* End with an anchor strip over the top of the foot, just proximal to the metatarsal heads, ensuring the toes can extend without the tape impeding toe motion. The final result is shown in *d*. A variation that includes an ankle stirrup support is shown in *e*.

▶ Video 2.7 demonstrates low dye strap taping as an alternative to the simple and x-arch taping procedures to support the longitudinal arch.

Longitudinal Arch Exercises

Flexibility exercises should include stretching the gastrocnemius and soleus muscles (figure 2.10). Patients can also stretch the arch by hyperextending the toes (figure 2.21).

Patients can strengthen the arch by focusing on the intrinsic muscles of the foot. Activities such as picking up marbles with the toes and using toe curls to draw a towel across the floor will isolate these muscles (figure 2.22).

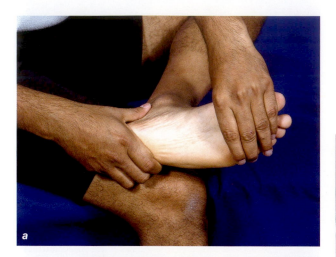

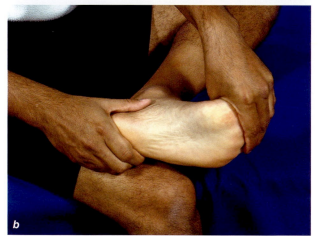

Figure 2.21   Stretch the plantar fascia by *(a)* grasping the ball of the foot and *(b)* extending the toes.

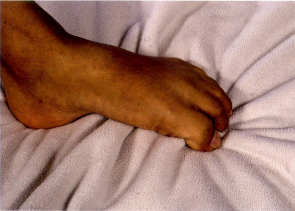

Figure 2.22   Strengthen the muscles that maintain the arch of the foot by curling the toes to grab a towel and sliding it across the floor. As the muscles become stronger, add weight to the towel to provide muscle resistance.

MORTON'S NEUROMA

This injury, also known as **plantar neuroma**, occurs when an interdigital nerve becomes inflamed where it passes between the heads of two metatarsal bones. Most often it affects the nerve between the third and fourth metatarsals, but it can involve other interdigital nerves. A fallen transverse arch or poor athletic footwear provides the mechanism for injury.

Transverse Arch Taping

Although athletic tape alone might provide adequate support for this injury, combining tape and a pad designed to support the transverse arch will be helpful. Use a commercially produced teardrop pad or a pad constructed from commercial padding and secure it in place with tape (figure 2.23). Completely resolving plantar neuroma may require more definitive medical treatment.

Transverse Arch Exercises

The longitudinal arch exercises may also be beneficial for this injury (see figures 2.21 and 2.22).

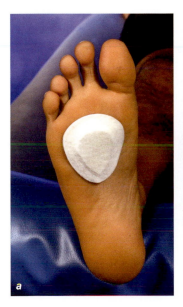 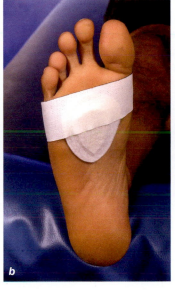 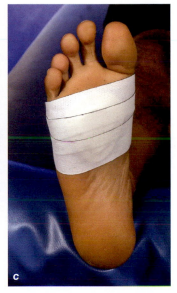

Figure 2.23 *(a)* Apply a commercially produced pad or cut a teardrop pad out of foam padding and *(b-c)* secure to the foot with tape. The tape should not be so tight that it restricts normal foot expansion during weight-bearing activity.

GREAT TOE SPRAINS

A sprain of the great toe, also known as turf toe, can be disabling. The injury usually results from hyperflexion or hyperextension of the first metatarsophalangeal joint. Patients competing on artificial turf have a higher incidence of injury because of the enhanced shoe–ground interface.

Sesamoiditis

A sesamoid bone is a small bone that develops within a tendon. In the foot, two sesamoids are found within the tendon of the flexor hallucis brevis. These bones help lift the first metatarsal, increasing the moment arm of the tendon to assist with plantar flexion of the first metatarsophalangeal joint.

Sesamoiditis is an inflammation of the bone and tendon that occurs from repetitive motion from activities such as running. The condition is more prevalent among young active adults with risk factors being the presence of pes cavus foot structure, ankle equinus, plantar flexed first ray, and large-sized sesamoid bones.

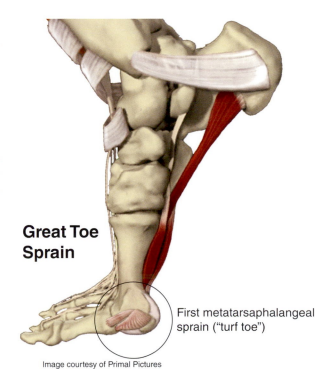

Great Toe Sprain

First metatarsaphalangeal sprain ("turf toe")

Image courtesy of Primal Pictures

Pain is often the first symptom reported and the condition is often treated conservatively to start. Treatment may include supportive great toe taping, and, in more severe cases, immobilization with a walking boot and reduced weight-bearing.

Great Toe Taping

Determine if hyperflexion or hyperextension produces the patient's discomfort (figure 2.24). Begin the procedure by applying anchor strips around the midfoot and the great toe. Then, depending on the mechanism of injury, place longitudinal strips along the dorsal surface to prevent hyperflexion or along the plantar surface to prevent hyperextension (figure 2.25). In some cases, strips of tape on both the dorsal and plantar surfaces may be necessary. Some patients may prefer elastic tape for this procedure. The taping procedure can be supplemented with a modified metatarsal bar (figure 2.26) that decreases load on the first metatarsophalangeal joint (MTP) by distributing pressure over the second through fifth MTP joints. You may also purchase steel-plate shoe inserts to use with the tape (figure 2.27).

 Video 2.8 demonstrates how to determine if a sprain is the result of hyperextension or hyperflexion and how to limit these motions to protect the sprained great toe.

Great Toe Exercises

The stretching and strengthening exercises for the longitudinal arch (see figures 2.21 and 2.22), when directed specifically to the great toe, will help the patient recover from this injury.

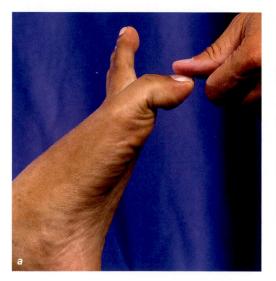 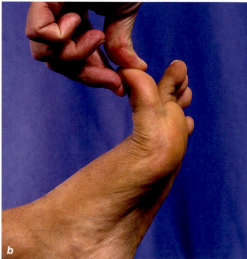

Figure 2.24   *(a)* Hyperflexion and *(b)* hyperextension of the great toe.

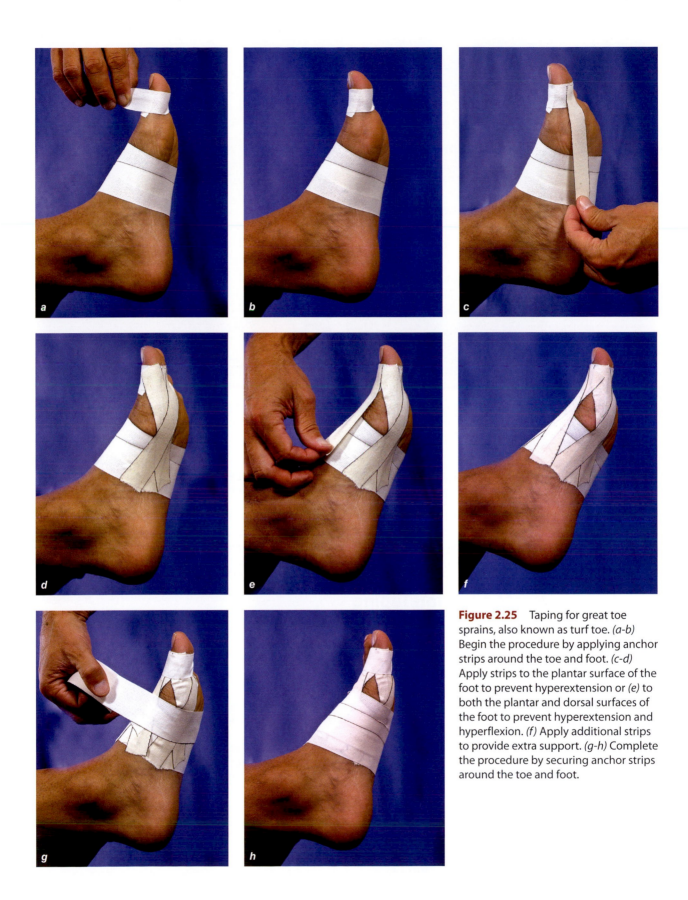

Figure 2.25 Taping for great toe sprains, also known as turf toe. *(a-b)* Begin the procedure by applying anchor strips around the toe and foot. *(c-d)* Apply strips to the plantar surface of the foot to prevent hyperextension or *(e)* to both the plantar and dorsal surfaces of the foot to prevent hyperextension and hyperflexion. *(f)* Apply additional strips to provide extra support. *(g-h)* Complete the procedure by securing anchor strips around the toe and foot.

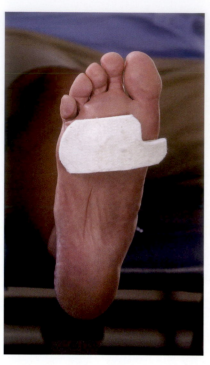

Figure 2.26 Application of metatarsal bar to reduce load on the first metatarsophalangeal joint.

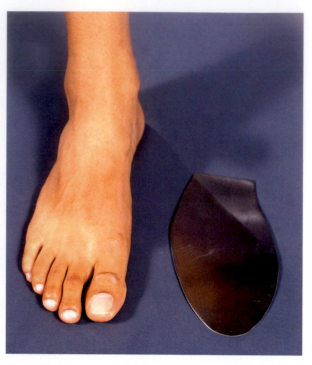

Figure 2.27 Use a steel-plate shoe insert to give additional support for turf toe by limiting flexion and extension of the great toe.

HEEL CONTUSIONS

A thick fat pad protects the calcaneus, or heel bone, on the plantar surface of the foot. Nevertheless, contusions of the calcaneus often cause pain and disable a physically active person. Either acute trauma or chronic stress can precipitate this injury. Improper footwear can also bruise the heel.

Heel Contusion Taping

Figure 2.28 illustrates taping that supports the calcaneus. You can also secure a pad to the heel with basketweave taping.

 Video 2.9 demonstrates a taping procedure to support and protect a bruised heel.

SHIN SPLINTS

The colloquial term **shin splints** refers to leg pain that arises from a variety of sources, such as arch strains, tendinitis, compartment syndrome, or stress fractures of the tibia or fibula. Seek the assistance of an experienced clinician to identify the source and mechanism of injury.

Arch Strains

A strain, or falling of the longitudinal arch, causes the tarsal bones of the foot to spread. The flattened foot can place undue stress where the extensor retinacula tie the anterior tendons to the leg, and the extra stress causes the patient to experience pain in the distal leg.

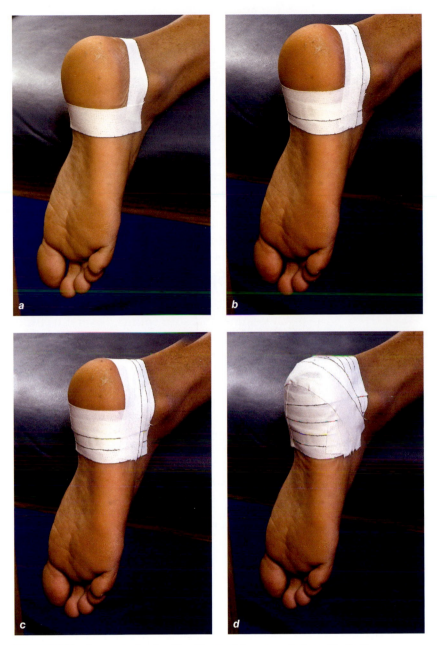

Figure 2.28   Support a bruised heel by applying tape designed to limit move-ment of the fat pad of the heel or to hold a protective pad in place. *(a)* Begin the procedure by applying anchor strips behind and below the heel. *(b-c)* Overlap strips in a weave pattern until you *(d)* completely cover the heel.

Tendinitis

Tendinitis may occur in any of the tendons that cross the ankle, but the posterior tibial tendon receives the greatest number of injuries. Running on uneven or banked surfaces that place one ankle in continuous eversion will precipitate injury. A hyper-pronated foot could also contribute to the injury mechanism.

Compartment Syndrome

The tibia, fibula, and superficial fascia of the leg create a compartment through which the anterior muscles, the deep peroneal nerve, a vein, and an artery traverse. When the anterior muscles swell, they create chronic anterior compartment syndrome, producing leg pain and numbness that radiate into the foot.

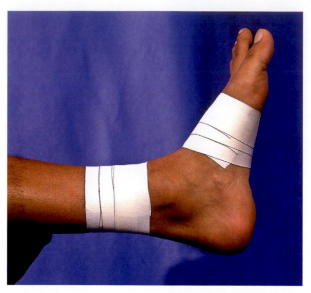

Figure 2.29 Taping procedure for shin splints caused by a weakened or fallen longitudinal arch. The procedure combines simple arch taping with reinforcement of the ankle retinacula. The retinacula secure the anterior tendons of the leg.

Stress Fractures

Stress fractures to the tibia or fibula are a disruption to the **periosteum** and commonly occur in patients who undergo prolonged periods of running. No taping procedure will help the symptoms associated with a stress fracture. The patient usually requires 6 weeks of rest before the symptoms resolve.

Shin Splint Taping

A haphazard taping approach often prevails in the treatment of shin splints. Several techniques exist to remedy leg pain. If the pain occurs because of a fallen longitudinal arch, the patient may find relief from simple arch taping combined with two or three strips placed around the distal leg to support the extensor retinacula (figure 2.29). A closed basketweave designed to limit eversion aids posterior tibial tendinitis. Patients have also reported relief from compression taping rather than from a procedure that supports the involved musculature (figure 2.30). No type of taping is likely to alleviate the effects of compartment syndrome or stress fractures.

 Video 2.10 demonstrates the application of tape to the anterior leg to support shin splints.

Shin Splint Exercises

The stretching and strengthening exercises for the ankle (see figures 2.10 and 2.11) and longitudinal arch (see figures 2.21 and 2.22) can also be effective in decreasing leg pain. Have the patient give special attention to achieving a balance between the strength of the anterior and posterior leg muscles. The patient should also use high-quality footwear.

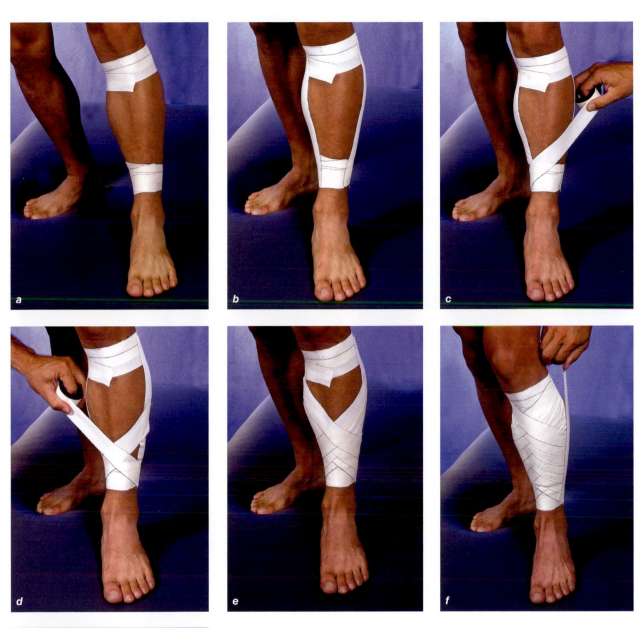

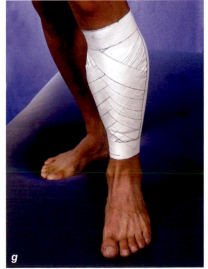

Figure 2.30 Apply tape to the anterior leg to support shin splints. Begin the procedure with *(a)* proximal and distal and *(b)* medial and lateral anchor strips. Apply tape in an oblique direction pulling *(c)* medial to lateral and *(d)* lateral to medial *(e)* in an overlapping fashion. Completely cover the anterior aspect of the leg. *(f)* Apply medial and lateral anchor strips to *(g)* complete the procedure.

FOOT ORTHOTICS

Orthotics can treat many of the injuries described in this chapter. Figure 2.31 shows an **orthotic** that you can easily mold and send to the manufacturer for fabrication; other orthotics require a plaster cast. Prescribe orthotics wisely because they are expensive. Have an experienced clinician carefully evaluate the foot and lower-extremity biomechanics before recommending foot orthotics. A multitude of approaches exist for the molding and fabrication of orthotics.

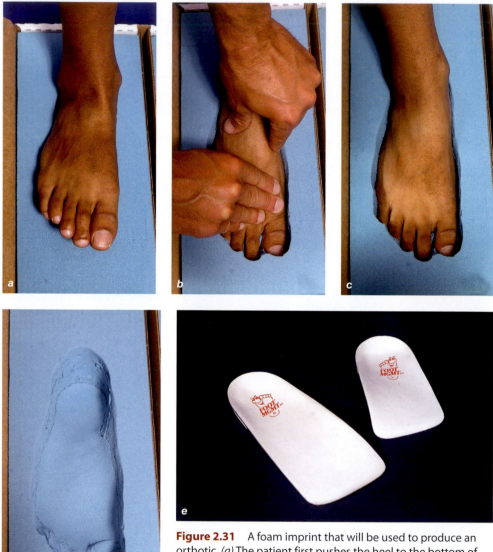

Figure 2.31 A foam imprint that will be used to produce an orthotic. *(a)* The patient first pushes the heel to the bottom of the foam, and *(b)* then the athletic trainer pushes the forefoot and toes to the bottom of the foam *(c)* to make an imprint of the entire foot. *(d)* Send the impression to the manufacturer for fabrication of *(e)* the orthotic.

FRACTURES OF THE FOOT AND ANKLE

The following sections discuss specifics related to fractures of the foot and ankle as well as methods for immobilizing these types of fractures.

Fifth Metatarsal Fractures

Fractures of the fifth metatarsal are the most common foot fractures and account for 45% to 70% of all metatarsal fractures. These injuries often occur in young males and result from physical activity and sports participation. Fifth metatarsal fractures are classified according to their location on the bone as avulsion, Jones, and mid-shaft (stress), moving proximal to distal.

Avulsion fractures occur at the base of the fifth metatarsal near the insertion of the peroneus brevis tendon. The acute mechanisms responsible for fifth metatarsal avulsion fractures include falling from a height or twisting the ankle when the foot is fixed, causing tension along the peroneus brevis tendon. Jones fractures occur proximal to the base of the fifth metatarsal between the diaphysis and metaphysis. The common mechanism of injury for an acute Jones fracture is a vertical or mediolateral force on the bone while the foot is plantar flexed and weight is shifted laterally. Mid-shaft or stress fractures result from a sudden increase in activity, repetitive motion, and chronic overloading of the bone during physical activity.

With an acute injury, patients will often complain about pain around the fifth metatarsal and the inability to bear weight. The foot may be swollen and discolored and pain is often present upon palpation of the metatarsal. Clinicians often use the Ottawa Foot Rules to determine the need for radiographic imaging. Conservative treatment is often used first with the foot being immobilized with a cast or splint. Operative treatment is only considered when there is bone displacement of more than 3 to 4 millimeters.

Mid-shaft or stress fractures present with initial complaints of pain only during activity; however, this may progress to an achy pain once activity has subsided. Patients may also complain of some swelling and discoloration if the stress fracture remains untreated and the patient continues weight-bearing activity. A reduction in activity along with immobilization is often the first-line treatment for stress fractures.

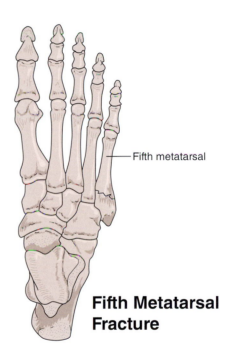

Fifth metatarsal

Fifth Metatarsal Fracture

Malleolar Fractures

Fractures can occur to both the medial malleolus and the lateral malleolus, with the rate of injury to the lateral malleolus occurring more often. Posterior malleolus fractures are also a concern and defined as a fracture to the posterior rim of the distal tibia. The mechanism of injury for a malleolar fracture is a forceful combined movement of inversion–internal rotation (lateral) or eversion–external rotation (medial). These fractures often occur in combination with associated ligamentous injury; therefore, treatment is usually dictated by the amount of instability in the joint.

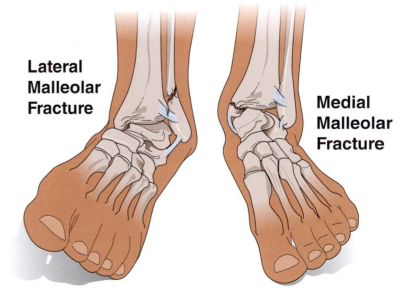

Lateral Malleolar Fracture

Medial Malleolar Fracture

Stable lateral malleolar fractures are typically managed conservatively with a cast application for 6 to 8 weeks with the patient non-weight bearing for 3 weeks and progressively increasing weight bearing after that time. In contrast, medial malleolar fractures often have associated deltoid ligament injury and may include fracture to the lateral or posterior malleoli. Non-displaced medial malleolar fractures can also be treated conservatively with a short leg cast that extends to the knee. Application of the cast should provide adequate control over rotation to ensure appropriate alignment during the healing process.

Methods for Immobilizing the Fractured Foot and Ankle

Immobilization of the fractured foot and ankle can be accomplished with splints or casts such as a posterior splint (figure 2.32), non-weight-bearing short leg cast (figure 2.33), and weight-bearing short leg cast (figure 2.34).

 Video 2.11 demonstrates the application of a posterior leg splint.

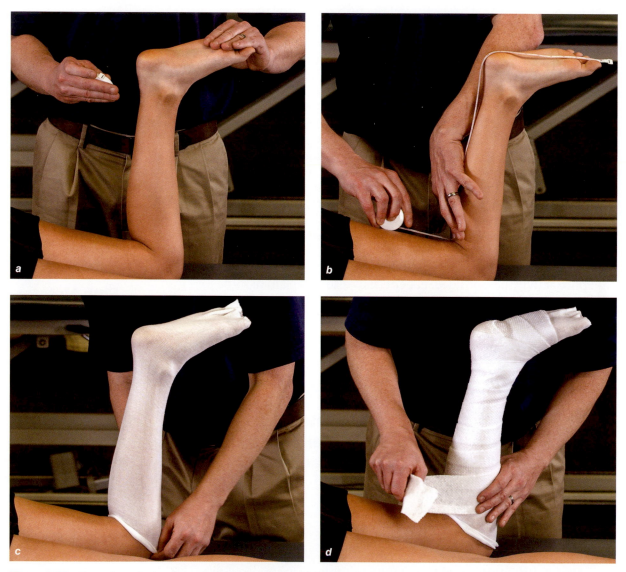

Figure 2.32   Posterior splinting procedure applied to immobilize the foot and ankle. *(a)* Position the foot and ankle in the functional position, which is 0° of dorsiflexion. *(b)* Measure 4 inches (10 cm) beyond the base of the popliteal fossa and 4 inches (10 cm) beyond the metatarsal heads to determine the amount of stockinette needed. *(c)* Apply the stockinette. *(d)* Beginning at the metatarsal heads, roll the cast padding circumferentially from distal to proximal ending at the base of the popliteal fossa.   *(continued)*

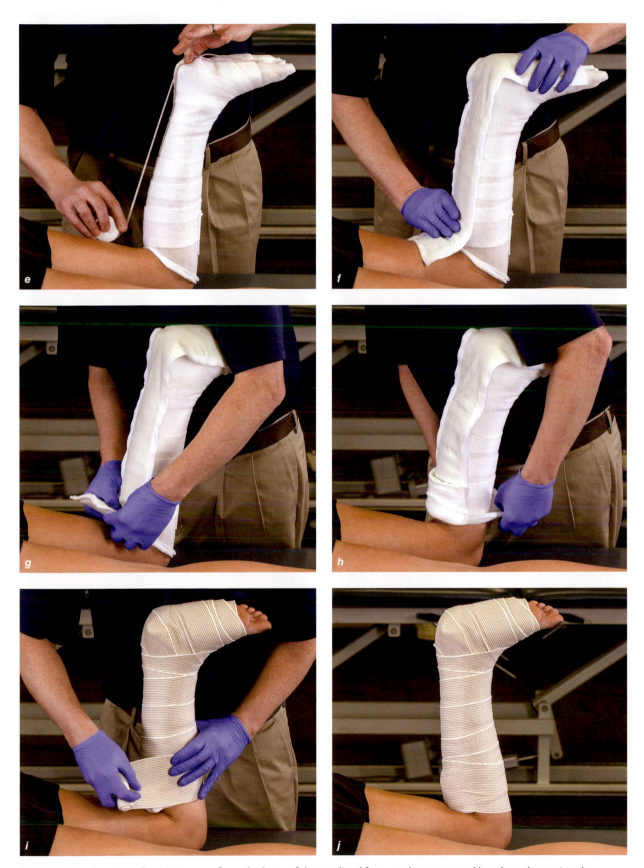

Figure 2.32 *(continued)* *(e)* Measure from the base of the popliteal fossa to the metatarsal heads to determine the length of the splint. *(f)* Starting at the metatarsal heads, position the posterior splint against the plantar surface of the foot and posterior aspect of the leg. *(g)* Fold down any excess splint material at the knee. *(h)* Fold the stockinette and cast padding over the ends of the fiberglass splint. *(i)* Starting distally, secure the splint in place with an elastic wrap. *(j)* Completed posterior splint.

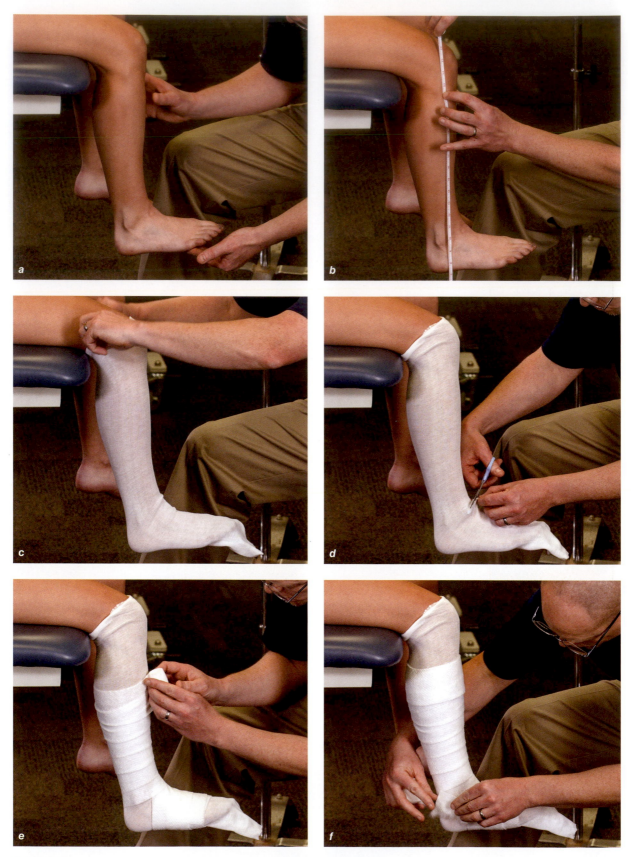

Figure 2.33 Non-weight-bearing short leg cast to immobilize the foot and ankle. *(a)* Position the foot and ankle in the functional position, which is 0° of dorsiflexion. *(b)* Measure 4 inches (10 cm) beyond the tibial tubercle and 4 inches (10 cm) beyond the metatarsal heads to determine the amount of stockinette needed. *(c)* Apply the stockinette, and *(d)* cut a slit in the stockinette across the front part of the ankle to eliminate any folds. *(e)* Beginning at the metatarsal heads, roll the cast padding circumferentially from distal to proximal, overlapping by 50% to end at the tibial tubercle. Do not cover the heel at this time. *(f)* Apply extra padding to protect the malleoli.   *(continued)*

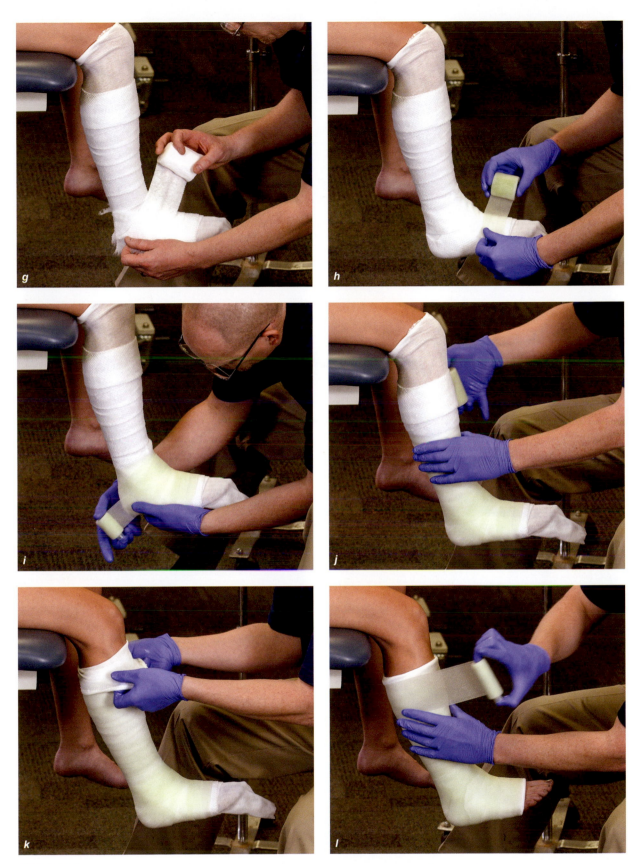

Figure 2.33 *(continued)* *(g)* Cast padding should now be applied to the heel. *(h)* Starting at the metatarsal heads, begin applying the fiberglass from distal to proximal, overlapping the previous layer by 50%. *(i)* Initially close in the foot and ankle with fiberglass, *(j)* followed by the lower leg. *(k)* Fold down the stockinette and *(l)* secure the ends of the stockinette with the final layers of fiberglass. *(continued)*

 Video 2.12 demonstrates the application of a non-weight-bearing short leg cast.

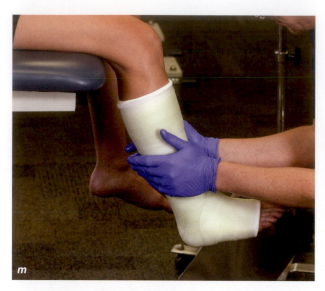

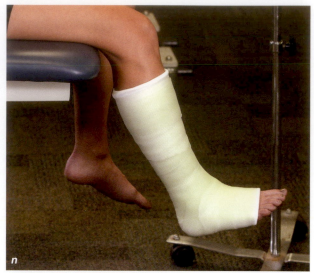

Figure 2.33 *(continued)* *(m)* Using the palm and heel of your hand, mold the casting material as needed. *(n)* Completed non-weight-bearing short leg cast.

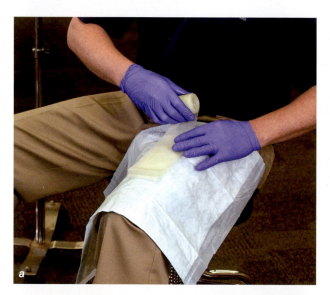

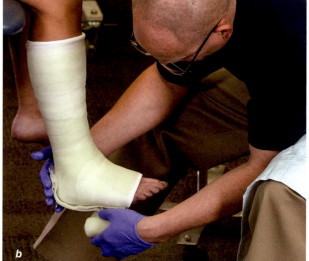

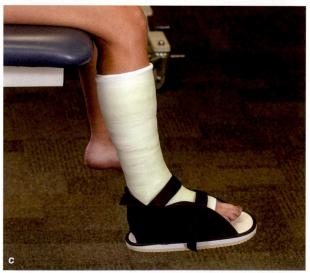

Figure 2.34 To create a weight-bearing short leg cast, extra fiberglass reinforcement needs to be applied to the plantar aspect of the foot and the heel. *(a)* Begin by folding the fiberglass casting material on itself to create a thickness of four to six layers. *(b)* Secure the extra fiberglass in place with an additional layer of fiberglass. *(c)* Make sure the patient wears a cast shoe to protect the cast.

Video 2.13 demonstrates the application of a weight-bearing short leg cast.

Splinting will be utilized for acute injuries until the post-traumatic swelling has resolved and any open wounds have healed. Based on the location of the fracture, the fracture alignment, and the amount of fracture healing that has taken place, the supervising physician will determine if the patient should be placed in a non-weight-bearing short leg cast or a weight-bearing short leg cast.

 Visit the web resource for checklists and video clips related to topics discussed in this chapter.

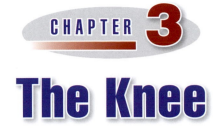
The Knee

The articulation of the distal femur and the proximal tibia forms the knee. The proximal tibia and fibula also create a joint that you will find more relevant to normal ankle inversion and eversion than knee movement. The gliding action of the patella in the intercondylar fossa of the femur creates the patellofemoral articulation, a region essential to normal knee function.

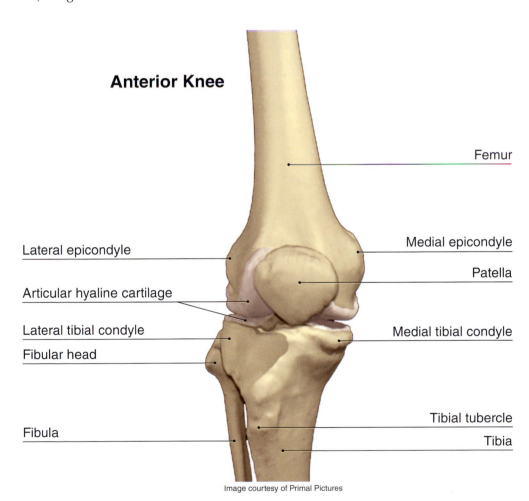

Anterior Knee

Femur

Lateral epicondyle

Medial epicondyle

Patella

Articular hyaline cartilage

Lateral tibial condyle

Medial tibial condyle

Fibular head

Tibial tubercle

Fibula

Tibia

Image courtesy of Primal Pictures

Knee movements include flexion and extension (figure 3.1). The knee is a modified hinge joint because the tibia internally rotates during flexion and externally rotates during extension.

Several ligaments stabilize the relatively shallow articulation between the femur and the tibia. The medial collateral ligament, also known as the tibial collateral ligament, supports the medial aspect of the knee by checking excess **valgus** displacement. The

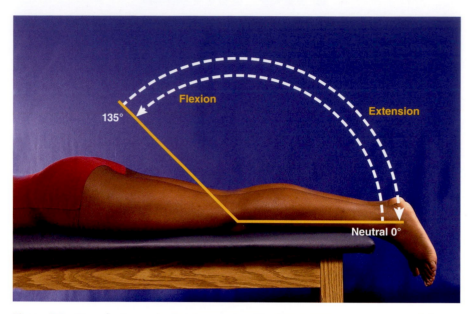

Figure 3.1   Knee flexion and extension ranges of motion.

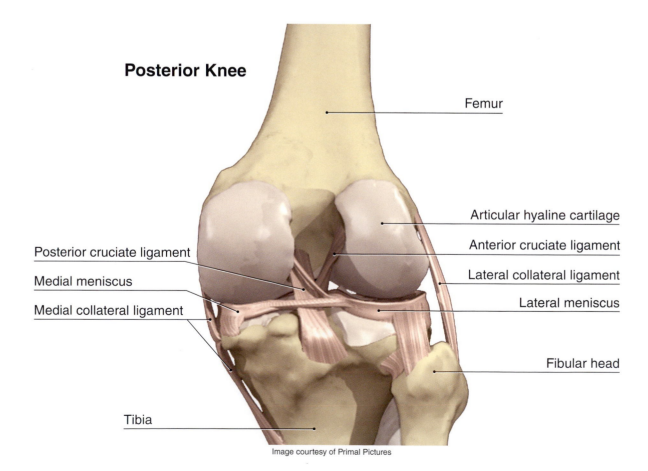

Image courtesy of Primal Pictures

lateral collateral ligament, also called the fibular collateral ligament, stabilizes the lateral aspect of the knee by preventing excess **varus** displacement.

The anterior and posterior cruciate ligaments cross within the knee joint. The **anterior cruciate ligament** prevents the anterior displacement of the tibia from the femur; the **posterior cruciate ligament** checks posterior displacement. Because the cruciate ligaments prevent rotary instabilities, their injury frequently causes either anterior-lateral or anterior-medial rotary instability.

Anterior-lateral instability occurs when the lateral tibial condyle slips forward. Anterior-medial instability results when the medial tibial condyle slips forward. All these rotational instabilities disable physically active people.

The intra-articular cartilage, the **menisci**, deepens the articulation and protects the joint surfaces of the tibia and femur. The medial meniscus has an oval shape and firmly attaches to the tibia and the medial collateral ligament. In contrast, the lateral meniscus is more round and moves more freely; it does not attach to the lateral collateral ligament. Meniscal injuries are especially problematic because, as **avascular** cartilage, they rarely heal.

The knee extends through the contraction of the powerful **quadriceps femoris** muscles. These muscles include the rectus femoris, vastus medialis, vastus intermedius, and vastus lateralis muscles. The fibers of the vastus medialis muscle attach to the

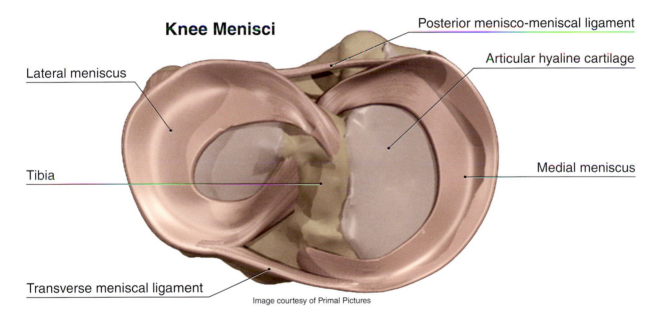

Knee Menisci

Posterior menisco-meniscal ligament

Articular hyaline cartilage

Lateral meniscus

Medial meniscus

Tibia

Transverse meniscal ligament

Image courtesy of Primal Pictures

medial border of the patella, and they are often called the vastus medialis oblique muscle. The quadriceps attach to the patella through the tendon of the quadriceps; this tendon passes over and around the patella and attaches to the tibia as the patellar tendon. These muscles suffer contusions during the patient's participation in contact sports.

The **hamstrings** muscle group produces knee flexion. These muscles include the medial semitendinosus and semimembranosus and the lateral biceps femoris; all these muscles experience strain during sprinting activities.

Several bursae exist around the knee to reduce the friction that the overlying muscle tendons create. These **bursae** include the suprapatellar, prepatellar, and the deep and superficial infrapatellar bursae. The suprapatellar directly communicates with the capsule of the knee joint. Excess fluid in this bursa represents significant swelling in the knee. The prepatellar bursa has a high contusion rate because of its anterior position to the joint.

Anterior Thigh Muscles

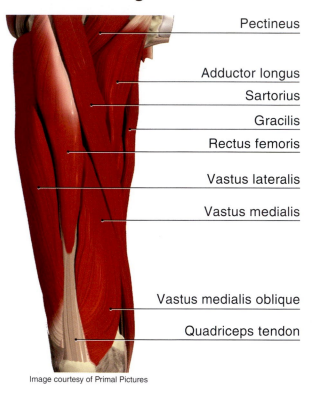

Pectineus

Adductor longus

Sartorius

Gracilis

Rectus femoris

Vastus lateralis

Vastus medialis

Vastus medialis oblique

Quadriceps tendon

Image courtesy of Primal Pictures

Posterior Thigh Muscles

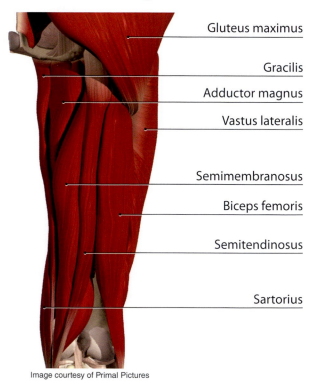

Gluteus maximus

Gracilis

Adductor magnus

Vastus lateralis

Semimembranosus

Biceps femoris

Semitendinosus

Sartorius

Image courtesy of Primal Pictures

Key Knee Palpation Landmarks

Medial Aspect
- Medial collateral ligament
- Medial joint line
- Medial meniscus

Lateral Aspect
- Lateral collateral ligament
- Lateral joint line
- Lateral meniscus

Anterior Aspect
- Quadriceps tendon
- Patella
- Patellar tendon

Posterior Aspect
- Popliteal fossa
- Biceps femoris tendon
- Semitendinosus tendon
- Semimembranosus tendon

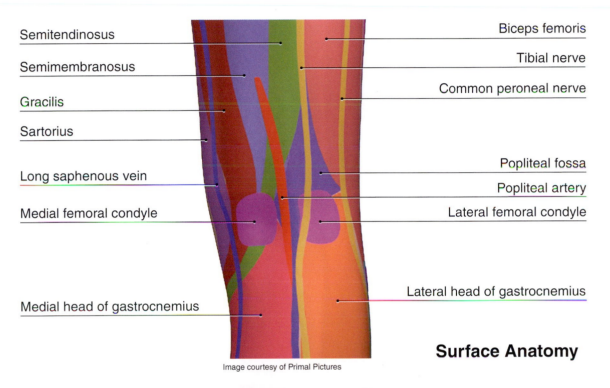

Semitendinosus

Semimembranosus

Gracilis

Sartorius

Long saphenous vein

Medial femoral condyle

Medial head of gastrocnemius

Biceps femoris

Tibial nerve

Common peroneal nerve

Popliteal fossa

Popliteal artery

Lateral femoral condyle

Lateral head of gastrocnemius

Surface Anatomy

Image courtesy of Primal Pictures

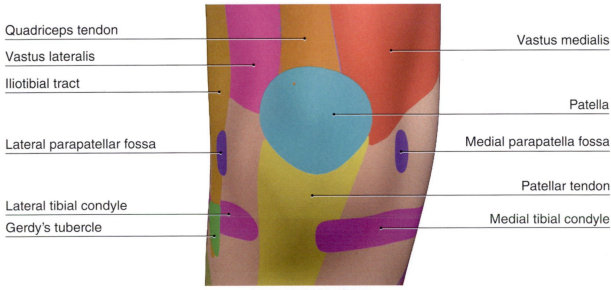

Quadriceps tendon

Vastus lateralis

Iliotibial tract

Lateral parapatellar fossa

Lateral tibial condyle

Gerdy's tubercle

Vastus medialis

Patella

Medial parapatella fossa

Patellar tendon

Medial tibial condyle

Image courtesy of Primal Pictures

COLLATERAL AND CRUCIATE LIGAMENT SPRAINS

The relative instability of the knee renders it highly vulnerable to sprains of the collateral and cruciate ligaments. Excessive valgus or varus forces sprain the medial and lateral collateral ligaments, respectively. You can expect to see fewer injuries to the lateral collateral ligament because the **contralateral** extremity protects the knee from varus forces. External forces directed at the outside of the knee produce valgus stress; they often implicate the anterior cruciate ligament and medial meniscus as well as the medial collateral ligament. Clinicians refer to this classic injury as the terrible triad.

Noncontact mechanisms often cause isolated injuries to the cruciate ligaments, particularly the anterior cruciate. Sudden deceleration, which occurs when the patient changes direction or dismounts from a gymnastic apparatus, can produce an isolated rupture of the anterior cruciate ligament. An external force anteriorly directed to the back of the tibia will also injure the anterior cruciate ligament, just as a posteriorly directed force from the front of the knee can injure the posterior cruciate ligament.

**Medial Collateral
Ligament Rupture**

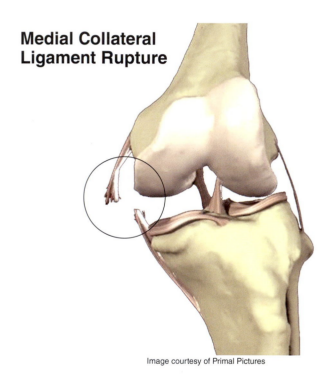

Image courtesy of Primal Pictures

**Anterior Cruciate
Ligament Rupture**

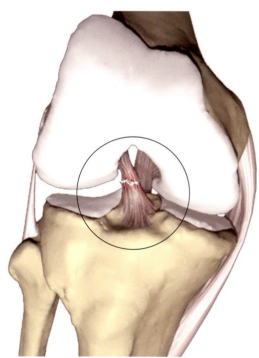

Image courtesy of Primal Pictures

Knee Sprain Taping

Figure 3.2 illustrates how to tape the collateral and cruciate ligaments. Execute a slight flexion by placing a lift under the heel. Avoid using a tape roll for this lift because heel pressure will ruin the tape! As with the ankle, optimize the procedure by taping directly on shaved skin and using minimal underwrap. We recommend elastic tape. Begin by placing proximal and distal anchors and then apply, in an X pattern, successive interlocking strips over the medial and lateral collateral ligaments. For the patient with a cruciate ligament injury, tape a series of medial and lateral spiral strips to enhance anterior, posterior, and rotary support.

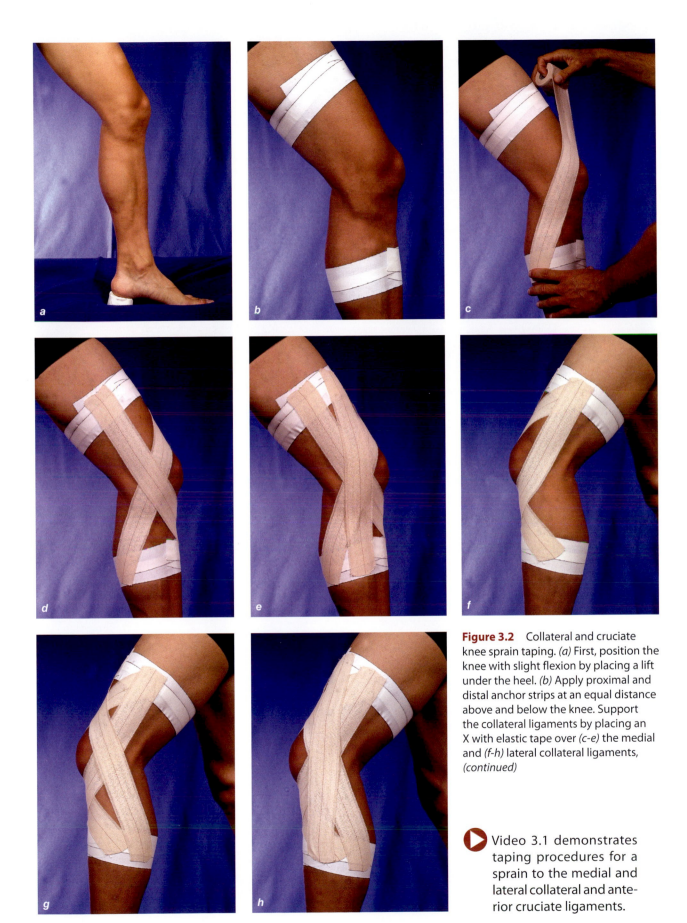

Figure 3.2 Collateral and cruciate knee sprain taping. *(a)* First, position the knee with slight flexion by placing a lift under the heel. *(b)* Apply proximal and distal anchor strips at an equal distance above and below the knee. Support the collateral ligaments by placing an X with elastic tape over *(c-e)* the medial and *(f-h)* lateral collateral ligaments, *(continued)*

Video 3.1 demonstrates taping procedures for a sprain to the medial and lateral collateral and anterior cruciate ligaments.

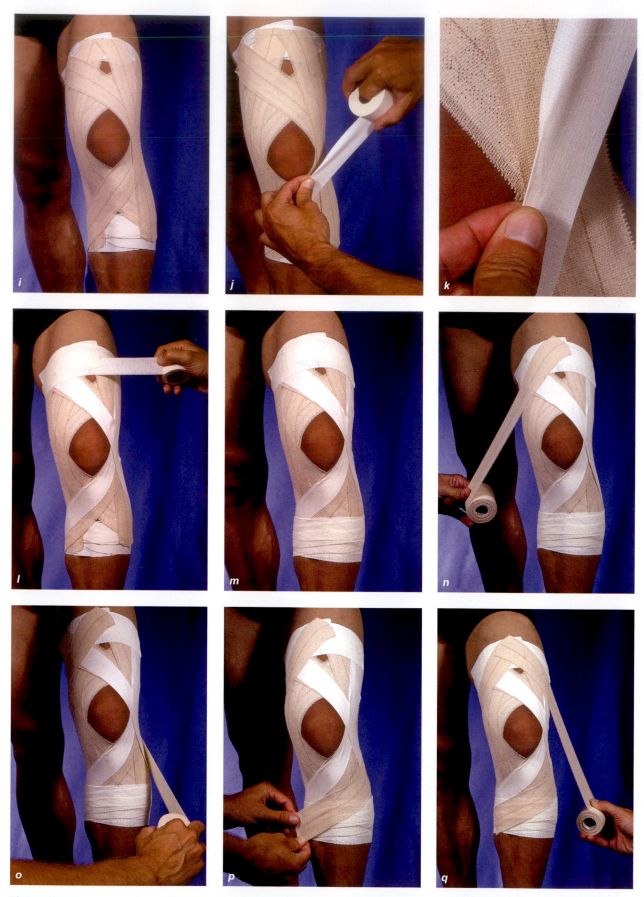

Figure 3.2 *(continued)* *(i)* leaving the patella open. *(j-k)* Reinforce the collateral strips by folding the edge of white tape and placing an additional X over the previously applied elastic tape. *(l-m)* Apply proximal and distal anchors to complete the collateral knee sprain taping. *(n-s)* For rotary instability that often results from injury to the anterior cruciate ligament, apply additional strips that begin on the anterior-proximal thigh, pass behind the knee, and end on the posterior leg. *(continued)*

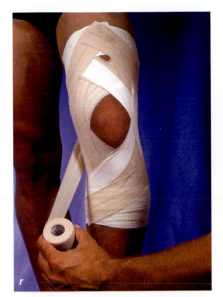
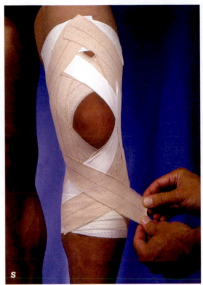
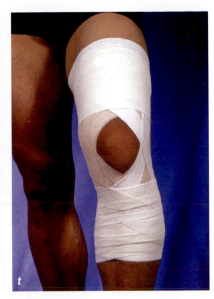

Figure 3.2 *(continued)* *(t)* Complete the procedure by enclosing the thigh and leg with elastic tape.

Knee Exercises

Injury-free, effective athletic participation requires the quadriceps and hamstrings muscles to have adequate strength and flexibility. Figure 3.3 illustrates static stretching exercises for these groups.

Strengthen the patient's quadriceps and hamstrings muscles by prescribing **open-chain exercises** with elastic bands (figure 3.4).

Figure 3.5 illustrates a strengthening device that provides progressive resistance for the knee.

Weight-bearing exercises from closed-chain positions will build the patient's strength and functional ability. The step-up (figure 3.6) and squat (figure 3.7) exercises are simple, yet effective, **closed-chain exercises.**

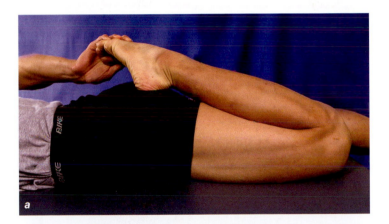

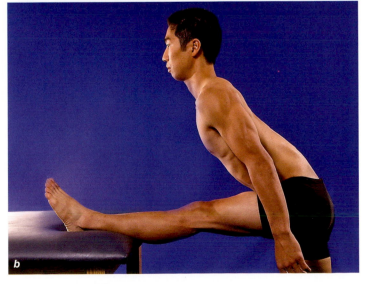

Figure 3.3 *(a)* Stretch the quadriceps muscle group by pulling the knee into flexion while the patient is lying prone. *(b)* Stretch the hamstrings by flexing the hip while maintaining knee extension. Note how the patient holds the back in a flattened position to ensure optimal isolation of the hamstrings muscles.

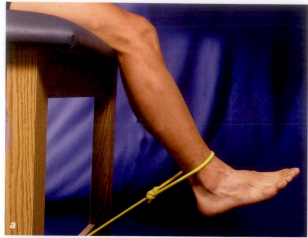

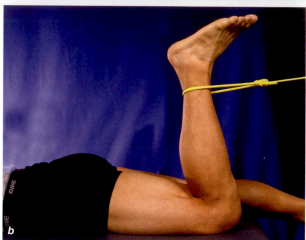

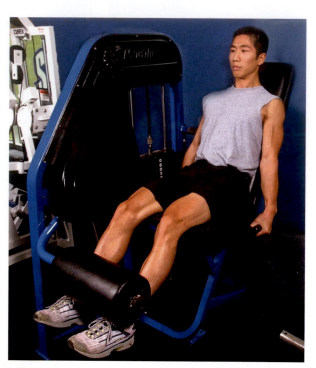

Figure 3.4 *(a)* Strengthen the quadriceps by resisting knee extension while the patient is seated. *(b)* Strengthen the hamstrings muscle group by providing resistance to knee flexion while the patient is lying prone.

Figure 3.5 Strengthen the quadriceps and hamstring muscles with a commercially available resistance device.

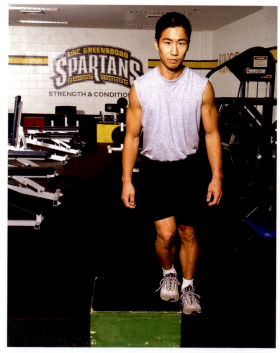

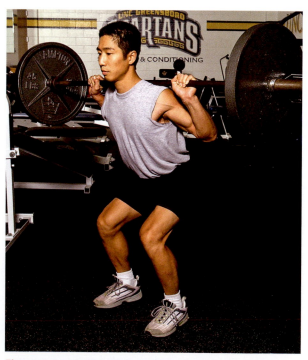

Figure 3.6 The step-up is an excellent example of a closed-chain exercise that incorporates the quadriceps as a knee extensor and the hamstrings as a hip extensor.

Figure 3.7 Closed-chain squat exercise for the knee extensor and hip extensor muscles.

KNEE BRACES

Knee braces fall into three categories: preventive, rehabilitative, and functional.

Preventive Braces

Preventive braces guard the knee from injury during athletic participation by protecting the medial collateral ligament from excessive valgus force. Speculation abounds concerning the potential of this brace to reduce injury to the medial col-

lateral ligament, and these braces are used far less frequently than they were in the past. Although patients, coaches, and athletic trainers offer anecdotal reports that the brace has saved the ligament, scientific research is less conclusive on the value of the preventive knee brace. We are wary of prescribing a preventive device because of its questionable clinical value and excessive cost.

Rehabilitative Braces

Rehabilitative braces protect the knee immediately after injury or surgery (figure 3.8). Clinicians can control the range of motion of the knee by adjusting dials on the medial and lateral aspects of the brace.

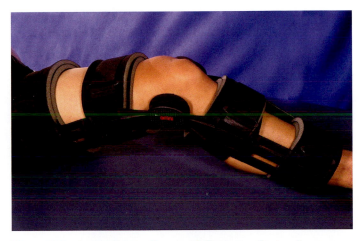

Figure 3.8   A rehabilitative brace with flexion and extension stops that can be used to control the degree of knee motion.

Functional Braces

Functional knee braces may be used on patients who experience rotary instability because of injury to the anterior cruciate ligament (figures 3.9 and 3.10). Some patients have found functional knee braces effective for their anterior cruciate ligament injuries; others require surgical reconstruction before returning to competition. Physicians may recommend or require a functional brace following surgical reconstruction of a knee with a deficient anterior cruciate ligament. The functional knee brace has the disadvantage of costing at least several hundred dollars.

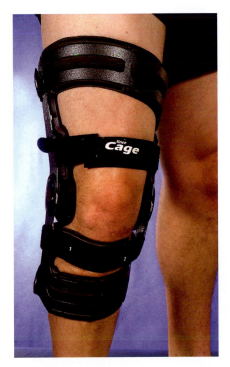

Figure 3.9   A functional knee brace to control rotary instability of the knee.

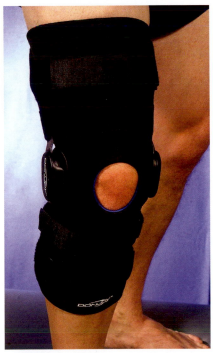

Figure 3.10   A functional knee brace with flexion and extension stops that can also control the amount of knee motion.

KNEE HYPEREXTENSION

Knee hyperextension occurs when an anteriorly directed or self-inflicted force causes the joint to extend beyond its normal anatomical limits. The cruciate ligaments, as well as the muscles and capsule located on the posterior aspect of the knee, may suffer damage.

Hyperextension Taping

Determine the degree of extension required to elicit knee discomfort. Place a lift under the heel to flex the patient's joint slightly. Make sure the patient maintains this position for the entire procedure. Begin by placing anchor strips around the thigh and calf and then apply successive strips in an X-pattern from the proximal to distal anchors over the posterior aspect of the joint. You may wish to complete the taping procedure by using an elastic wrap to enclose the knee (figure 3.11).

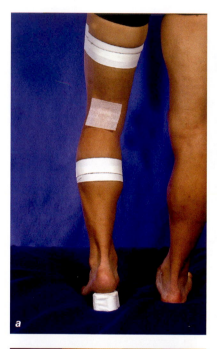
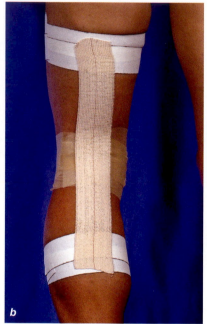
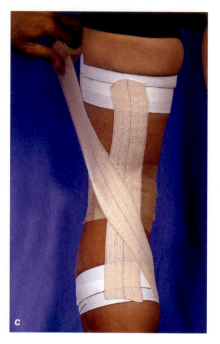

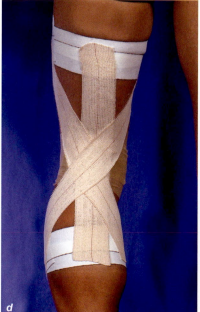
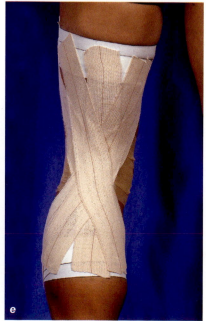

Figure 3.11   Begin knee hyperextension taping by placing a lift under the heel to flex the knee. *(a)* Protect the back of the knee with a pad and apply proximal and distal anchor strips. *(b)* Use elastic tape to apply a vertical strip and *(c-e)* then overlap with two strips, creating an X over the back of the knee.   *(continued)*

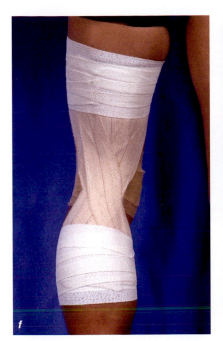
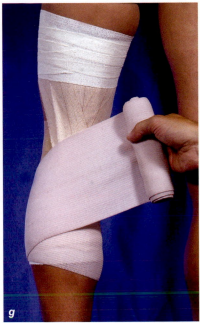
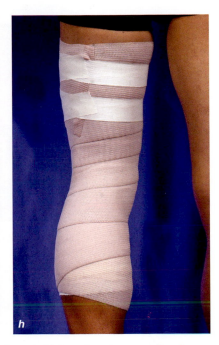

Figure 3.11 *(continued)* *(f)* Apply proximal and distal anchors to secure the procedure. *(g-h)* Complete the procedure by enclosing the knee in an elastic wrap.

 Video 3.2 demonstrates a taping procedure to limit extension in the hyperextended knee.

For a more rigid hyperextension limit that does not need to be reapplied more than once every few days, use strap taping instead (figure 3.12). It can be applied either standing or prone, maintaining the degree of knee flexion desired. The functional knee brace illustrated in figure 3.10 can also be used to limit knee extension, which can protect a knee from going into hyperextension. Figure 3.13 depicts how a range of motion block can be applied to a hinged knee brace in order to prevent hyperextension.

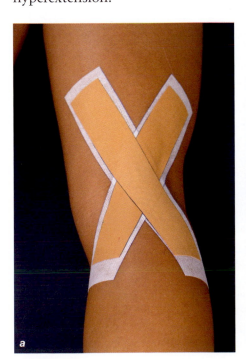
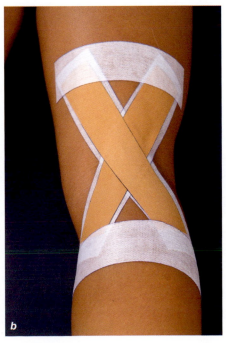

Figure 3.12 Strap taping a knee hyperextension block. *(a)* Place an X with underwrap and strapping tape in the center of the popliteal fossa while the patient is prone with the knee slightly flexed or fully extended. Avoid wrinkles with this application because it will feel uncomfortable when the patient flexes the knee. *(b)* Anchor strips can be placed on the hamstring and calf.

 Video 3.3 demonstrates using a strap taping block to limit knee hyperextension.

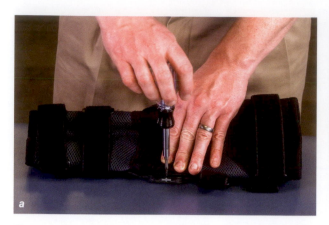
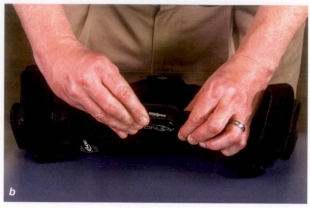

Figure 3.13   Applying a range of motion block to a hinged knee brace in order to prevent hyperextension. *(a)* Begin by removing the screws that hold in place the plastic guard that protects the hinges. *(b)* Insert the range of motion block on the front part of the hinge to protect the knee from hyperextending. The range of motion block will be secured in place by the screws that secure the plastic guard.

 Video 3.4 demonstrates inserting a range of motion block into a hinged knee brace.

Kinesiology taping also is an alternative for knee pain or swelling related to conditions such as patellar tendinitis, patellofemoral syndrome, quadriceps tendinitis, quadriceps strains, and knee arthritis when motion of the knee cannot be limited by tape (figure 3.14).

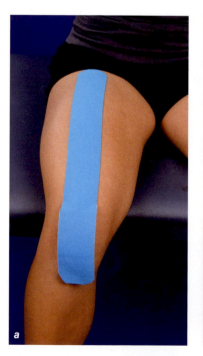
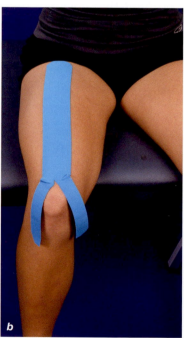
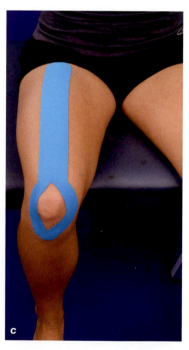

Figure 3.14   Kinesiology taping for anterior knee or quadriceps problems. *(a)* Measure a strip from the anterior inferior iliac spine (AIIS) or midthigh to distal to the patellar tendon. Cut edges round. With the patient sitting, start proximally on the thigh with a moderate pull to the tape when the knee is flexed to 90°; anchor it on the superior patella. *(b)* Cut a Y distal to this. *(c)* Maximally flex the knee and apply light tension surrounding the patella and anchor on the patellar tendon.

 Video 3.5 demonstrates kinesiology taping for anterior knee or quadriceps problems.

Hyperextension Exercises

Exercise should restore normal flexibility and strength of the hamstrings. The stretching and strengthening exercises for knee sprains (see figures 3.3 and 3.4) will accomplish this goal.

PATELLOFEMORAL JOINT PAIN

Physically active people commonly experience extensor mechanism pain arising from the patellofemoral articulation. Because this pain may result from numerous causes, an experienced clinician should carefully analyze the patient's condition. The injury mechanisms include a malalignment of the patella, an increased **quadriceps (Q) angle**, hyperpronation of the feet, or a weak vastus medialis oblique muscle.

Patellofemoral Taping

Provide patellofemoral support to displace the patella medially or realign it. Knee sleeves with lateral buttresses will supply medial displacement (figure 3.15), and the McConnell taping technique will realign the patella (figure 3.16). The taping procedure requires you to evaluate both the position of the patella and the patient's response to your treatment. Carefully analyze whether the taping relieves the patient's pain while he or she performs functional activities. McConnell taping, which requires a special tape that is more rigid than the nonelastic variety, is only one component of a complete patellofemoral treatment and rehabilitation program.

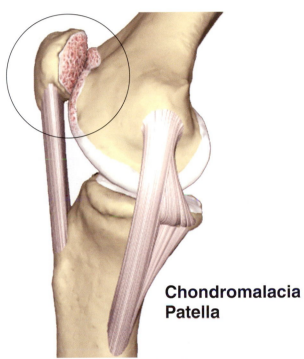

Chondromalacia Patella

Image courtesy of Primal Pictures

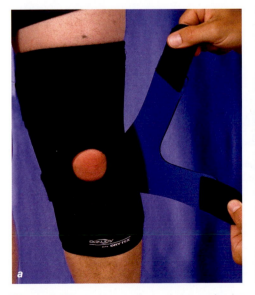 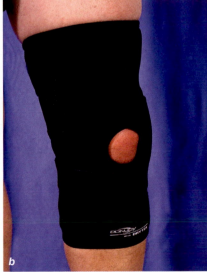

Figure 3.15 *(a-b)* Use a knee sleeve with a lateral buttress to facilitate normal tracking of the patella within the intercondylar fossa of the femur.

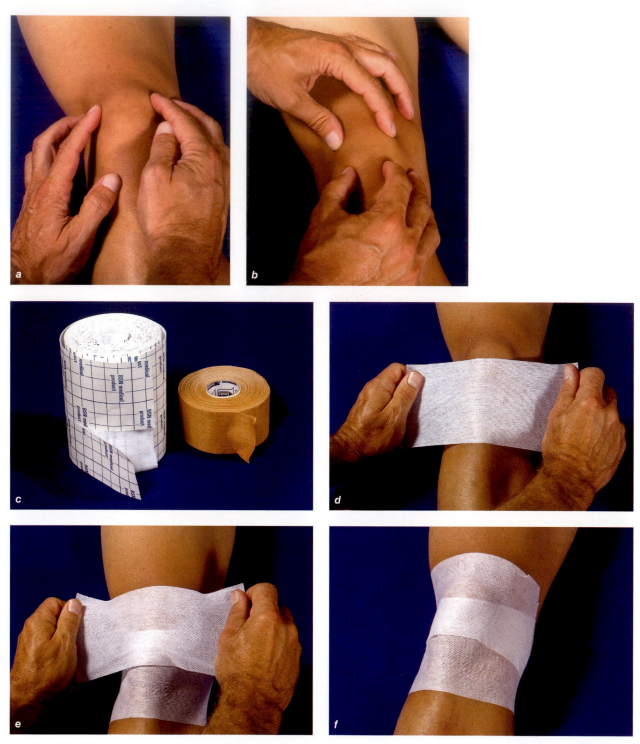

Figure 3.16 McConnell taping for a patient with patellofemoral pain. *(a-b)* Assess the patella for tilt and rotation positioning. *(c)* Use underwrap stretch and strapping tape for the taping procedure. *(d-f)* After shaving the knee, cover the patella with underwrap tape. *(continued)*

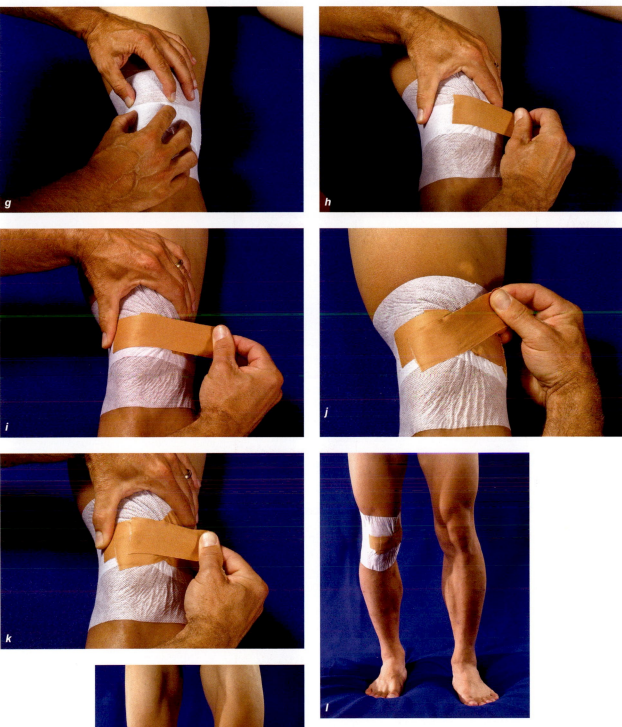

Figure 3.16 *(continued)* *(g)* Reassess for position. *(h)* Correct the tilt of the patella by applying a piece of strapping tape from the middle of the patella to the medial femoral condyle. *(i)* Correct the glide of the patella by applying the strapping tape from the lateral border of the patella and pulling medially to the medial femoral condyle. *(j)* Correct external rotation by applying strapping tape from the inferior pole (border) of the patella, pulling toward the opposite shoulder. *(k)* If the tilt of the patella is not correct, apply an additional tilt strip. *(l-m)* Reassess the patient for pain while he or she performs the functional activities that cause discomfort.

Video 3.6 demonstrates McConnell (strap) taping for patellofemoral pain.

Extensor Mechanism Exercises

The stretching exercises for knee sprains, which restore the normal flexibility of both the quadriceps and hamstrings muscles, will also help patients who experience patellofemoral pain. The patient should also strengthen the quadriceps muscles, although providing resistance to knee extension through the full range of motion of the joint may increase patellofemoral compression and aggravate the injury. Modify the quadriceps strengthening exercises for knee sprains to isolate the extension of the knee in its final 30° or find the range of motion through which the patient can exercise pain-free. Although not as effective as resisted knee extension, straight-leg raises will also exercise the quadriceps without significantly increasing patellofemoral compression (figure 3.17). If necessary, use **electrical muscle stimulation** or **biofeedback** to strengthen the vastus medialis oblique muscle—techniques that you will learn in your therapeutic exercise class.

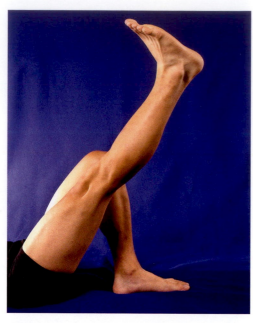

Figure 3.17   Use straight-leg raises to strengthen the muscles of the quadriceps without concomitant increases in patellofemoral compression.

 Visit the web resource for checklists and video clips related to topics discussed in this chapter.

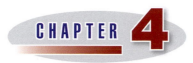
The Thigh, Hip, and Pelvis

The ball of the hip, the head of the femur, the socket, and the acetabulum of the pelvis create an extremely stable articulation.

The pelvic girdle contains two **innominate bones**, each possessing an ilium, a pubis, and an ischium. The pelvis protects the abdomen and serves as the point of attachment for many of the muscles acting on the hip and trunk.

Anterior Hip and Pelvis

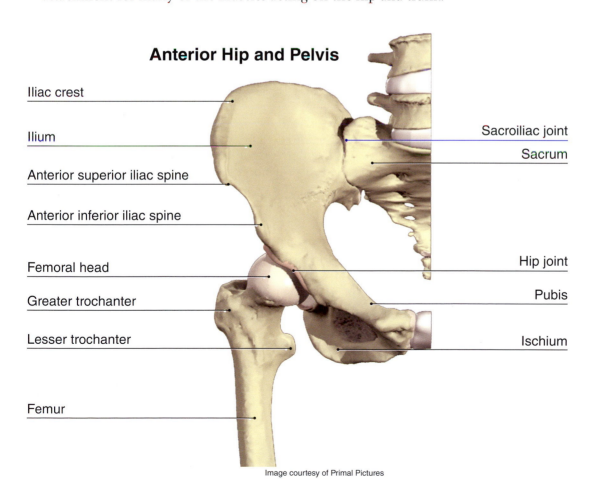

Iliac crest

Ilium

Anterior superior iliac spine

Anterior inferior iliac spine

Femoral head

Greater trochanter

Lesser trochanter

Femur

Sacroiliac joint

Sacrum

Hip joint

Pubis

Ischium

Image courtesy of Primal Pictures

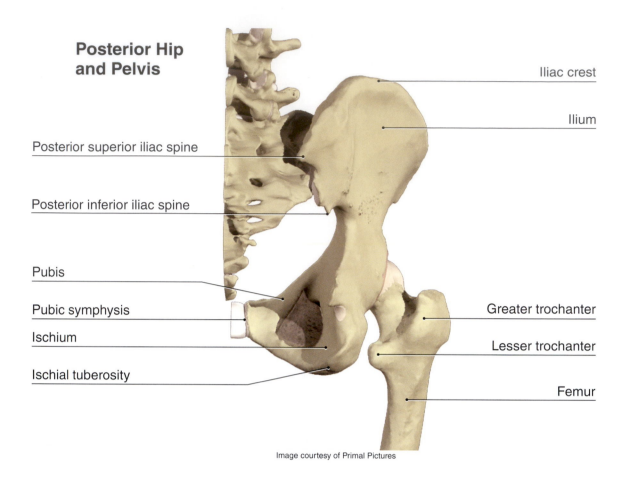

Posterior Hip and Pelvis

Iliac crest

Ilium

Posterior superior iliac spine

Posterior inferior iliac spine

Pubis

Pubic symphysis

Ischium

Ischial tuberosity

Greater trochanter

Lesser trochanter

Femur

Image courtesy of Primal Pictures

Hip joint movements include flexion and extension, abduction and adduction, medial and lateral rotation (figure 4.1), and **circumduction**.

A thick capsule and three major ligaments reinforce the hip joint. The anterior ligament is the iliofemoral, also called the Y-ligament; it checks excessive hip exten-

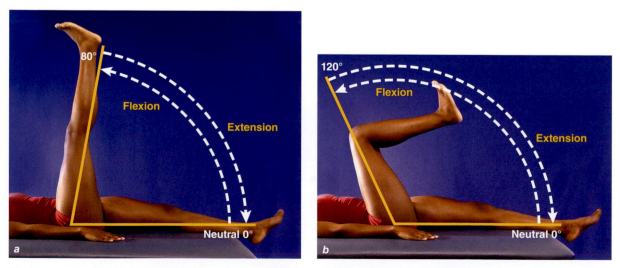

Figure 4.1   Hip flexion and extension ranges of motion with *(a)* knee extended and *(b)* flexed;   *(continued)*

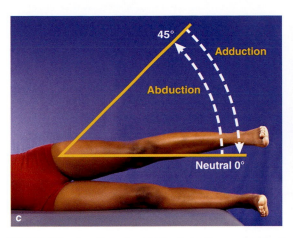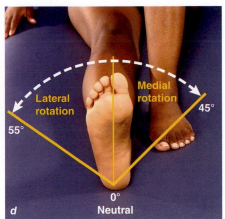

Figure 4.1 *(continued)* *(c)* hip abduction and adduction ranges of motion; *(d)* hip medial and lateral rotation ranges of motion.

sion. The medial ligament is the pubofemoral; it limits excess hip abduction. The posterior ligament is the ischiofemoral, which becomes taut during hip flexion. The depth of the hip joint, combined with its substantial capsular and ligament structures, contributes to the considerable stability of this joint.

Several muscle groups govern movement at this multidirectional joint. The iliopsoas and the rectus femoris muscles of the quadriceps produce flexion. Extension results from the contraction of the gluteus maximus and the three hamstrings muscles.

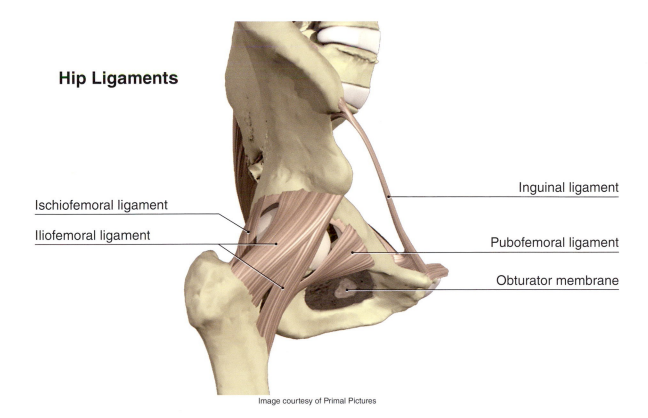

Hip Ligaments

Ischiofemoral ligament

Iliofemoral ligament

Inguinal ligament

Pubofemoral ligament

Obturator membrane

Image courtesy of Primal Pictures

Hip Rotator Muscles

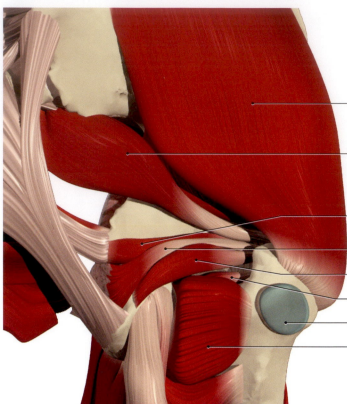

Gluteus medius

Piriformis

Gemellus superior

Obturator internus

Gemellus inferior

Obturator externus

Trochanteric bursa

Quadratus femoris

Image courtesy of Primal Pictures

Posterior Hip Muscles

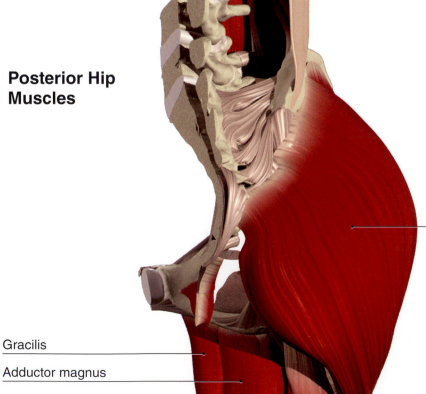

Gluteus maximus

Gracilis

Adductor magnus

Image courtesy of Primal Pictures

The gluteus medius and tensor fasciae latae muscles produce primary abduction, and the adductor magnus, longus, and brevis muscles cause adduction. The muscle group that includes the piriformis, gemellus superior and inferior, obturator internus and externus, and the quadratus femoris produces outward rotation. The tensor fasciae latae produce inward rotation.

HIP STRAINS

Hip muscle strains, or groin pulls, involve either the hip flexor muscles or the adductor muscle group. The patient usually overstretches or violently contracts the muscles. Lack of flexibility or strength, as well as inadequate preexercise warm-up, will precipitate strains.

Key Thigh, Hip, and Pelvis Palpation Landmarks

Anterior
► Rectus femoris muscle
► Vastus medialis muscle
► Vastus lateralis muscle
► Anterior superior iliac spine

Medial
► Adductor longus muscle
► Gracilis muscle
► Adductor magnus muscle

Lateral
► Iliac crest

Posterior
► Posterior superior iliac spine
► Ischial tuberosity
► Gluteus maximus muscle
► Biceps femoris muscle
► Semitendinosus muscle
► Semimembranosus muscle

Surface Anatomy

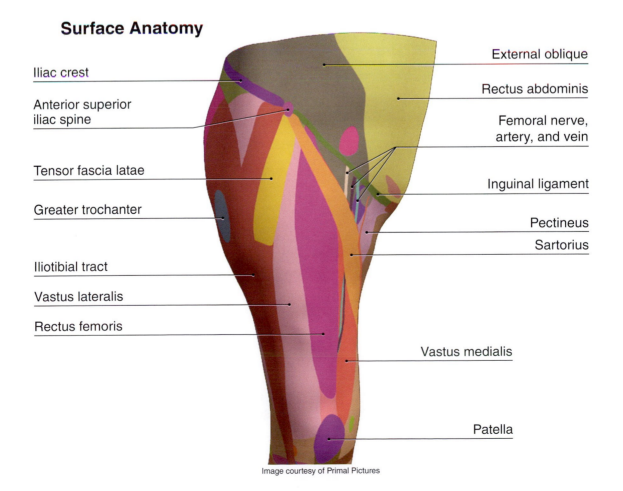

Iliac crest

Anterior superior iliac spine

Tensor fascia latae

Greater trochanter

Iliotibial tract

Vastus lateralis

Rectus femoris

External oblique

Rectus abdominis

Femoral nerve, artery, and vein

Inguinal ligament

Pectineus

Sartorius

Vastus medialis

Patella

Image courtesy of Primal Pictures

Hip Strain Taping

Support the hip muscles with an elastic bandage supplemented with elastic tape. Wrap the bandage around the thigh and hip in a **spica** pattern. Before treatment you should determine if the patient has damaged the hip flexor or adductor muscles. Examine for pain or weakness in these groups by using resistance to test hip flexion and adduction, in that order (figure 4.2). The affected muscle group will determine the direction in which you apply the hip spica.

When wrapping adductor muscles, have the patient internally rotate the hip. Place the wrap from a lateral to medial direction. Begin at midthigh and proceed to encircle the thigh and wind around the waist (figure 4.3, *a-h*). Use double-length elastic wrap, if available, and reinforce the wrap by tracing the pattern with elastic tape. Use a similar procedure to support the hip flexor muscles (figure 4.3, *i-o*), except begin with the hip in an externally rotated position and reverse the direction of the pull of the wrap. Before applying the wrap, place a lift under the heel of the extremity to shorten the hip flexors.

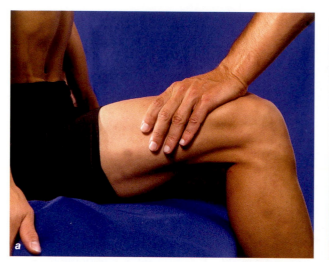
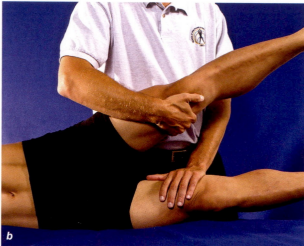

Figure 4.2 *(a)* Test the hip flexor muscles for strength by resisting the patient's efforts to flex the hip while seated. *(b)* Test the adductor muscles by having the patient lie on his or her left side. The patient then resists your efforts to abduct the right thigh.

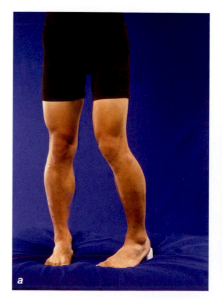
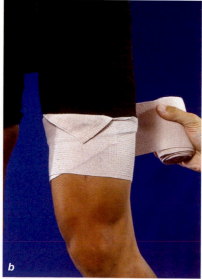
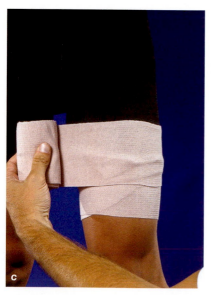

Figure 4.3 A hip spica with elastic wrap to support a strain of the adductor muscles. *(a)* Have the patient place the hip in an internally rotated position. *(b-c)* Apply an elastic wrap by pulling the thigh into internal rotation. Note how the elastic wrap folds over itself to lock it in place.   *(continued)*

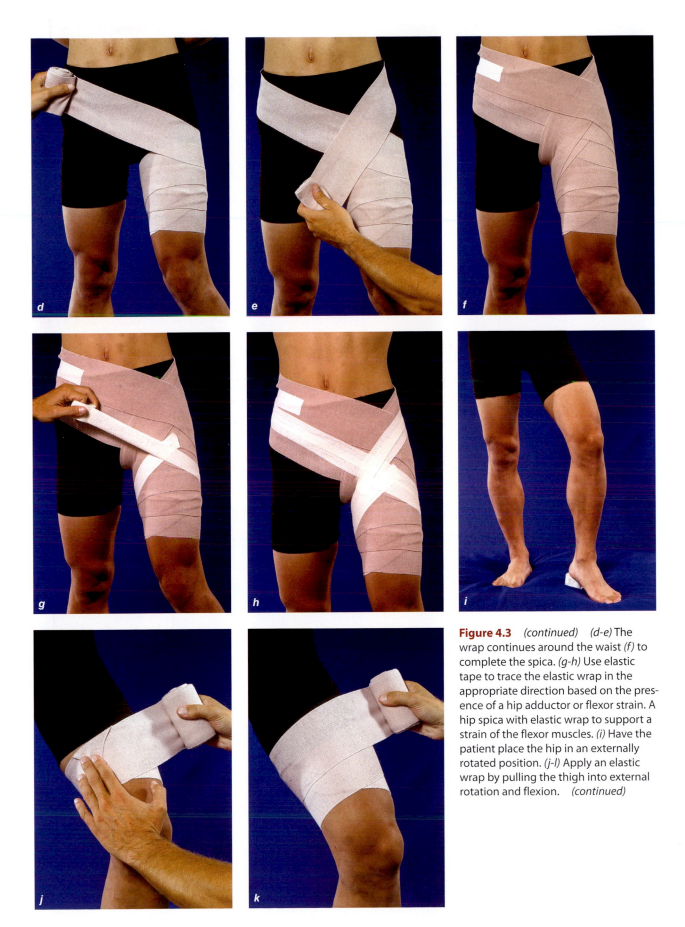

Figure 4.3 *(continued)* *(d-e)* The wrap continues around the waist *(f)* to complete the spica. *(g-h)* Use elastic tape to trace the elastic wrap in the appropriate direction based on the presence of a hip adductor or flexor strain. A hip spica with elastic wrap to support a strain of the flexor muscles. *(i)* Have the patient place the hip in an externally rotated position. *(j-l)* Apply an elastic wrap by pulling the thigh into external rotation and flexion. *(continued)*

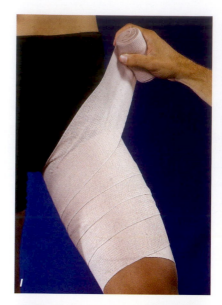

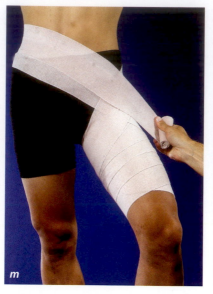

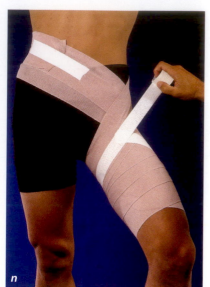

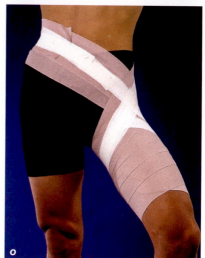

Figure 4.3 *(continued)* *(m)* The wrap continues around the waist to complete the spica. *(n-o)* Use elastic tape to trace the elastic wrap in the same direction as the elastic wrap.

Kinesiology taping of the hip (figure 4.4) can be used when motion of the hip cannot be limited and for pain related to iliotibial band friction syndrome, trochanteric bursitis, and hip arthritis.

 Video 4.1 demonstrates the application of a figure-eight (spica) wrap to support the hip adductor and hip flexor muscles.

 Video 4.2 demonstrates kinesiology taping for hip problems.

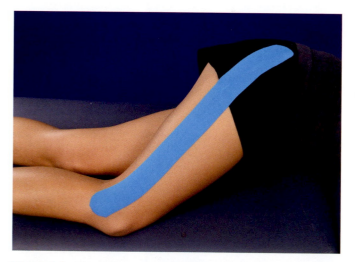

Figure 4.4 Kinesiology taping for hip problems. With the patient sidelying, measure a strip from superior to the iliac crest to the lateral knee. Flex the hip and adduct the leg to place the iliotibial band on stretch and apply the tape from the iliac crest to the distal leg with some tension.

Hip Exercises

The patient must maintain normal strength and flexibility in the hip muscles to prevent or treat strains. Figure 4.5 illustrates a static stretching exercise for the hip. Elastic bands can also supply resistance to strengthen the joint (figure 4.6). Because the rectus femoris of the quadriceps and all three hamstrings muscles act on the hip, the exercises for these groups are also appropriate (see chapter 3).

THIGH STRAINS

Strains occasionally occur to the quadriceps femoris muscles and more frequently to the hamstrings. The strain may result from overstretching, a violent contraction, or general muscle fatigue. For hamstrings strains, determine whether the injury involves the medial (semitendinosus and semimembranosus) or the lateral (biceps femoris) muscles. Isolate the medial and lateral hamstrings during muscle testing by rotating the leg internally and externally, respectively, during resisted knee flexion (figure 4.7).

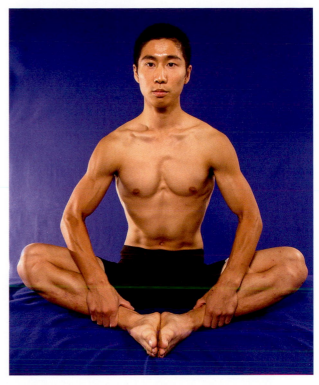

Figure 4.5 Stretching exercise for the hip.

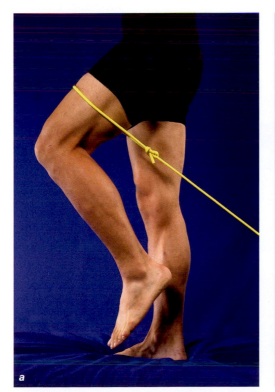
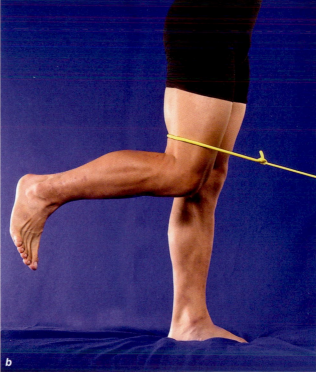

Figure 4.6 Strengthening exercises for (a) the hip flexor and (b) extensor muscles.

Thigh Strain Taping

Support the quadriceps (figure 4.8) and hamstrings (figure 4.9) muscles with an elastic wrap and, if necessary, supplement the wrap with elastic tape. Use a 4- or 6-inch-wide (10.2- or 15.2-cm-wide) elastic wrap to encircle the thigh. Cover the muscles both distal and proximal to the point of strain to provide optimal support. For a high strain, you may need to incorporate a hip spica to support the proximal muscle attachment. You can also use a taping procedure alone or in combination with an elastic wrap to support a thigh strain.

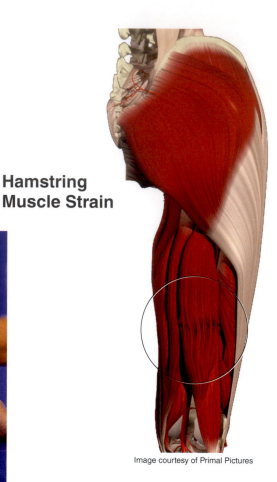

**Hamstring
Muscle Strain**

Image courtesy of Primal Pictures

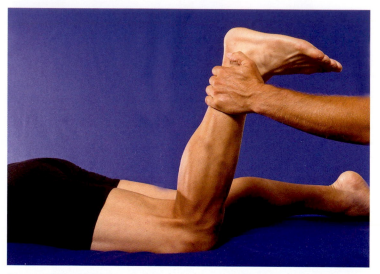

Figure 4.7 Test for hamstrings muscle strain. To isolate the medial hamstrings, resist knee flexion while internally rotating the leg. For isolation of the lateral hamstrings, resist knee flexion while externally rotating the leg.

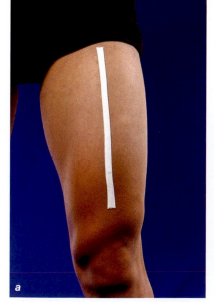 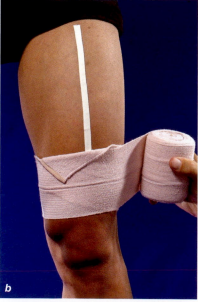 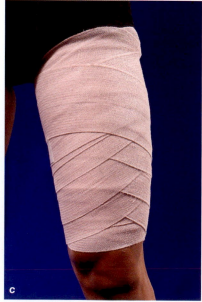

Figure 4.8 Elastic wrap to support a strain of the quadriceps muscles. *(a)* To prevent slipping of the wrap, apply tape adherent, or roll tape into a small strip and apply the roll to the thigh before applying the wrap. *(b-c)* Apply the wrap in a circular pattern around the thigh.   *(continued)*

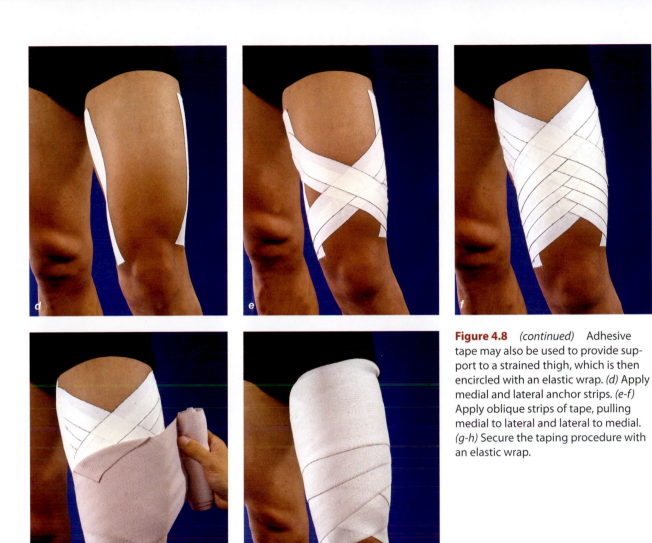

Figure 4.8 *(continued)* Adhesive tape may also be used to provide support to a strained thigh, which is then encircled with an elastic wrap. *(d)* Apply medial and lateral anchor strips. *(e-f)* Apply oblique strips of tape, pulling medial to lateral and lateral to medial. *(g-h)* Secure the taping procedure with an elastic wrap.

▶ Video 4.3 demonstrates the application of an elastic wrap and a taping procedure to support a quadriceps muscle strain.

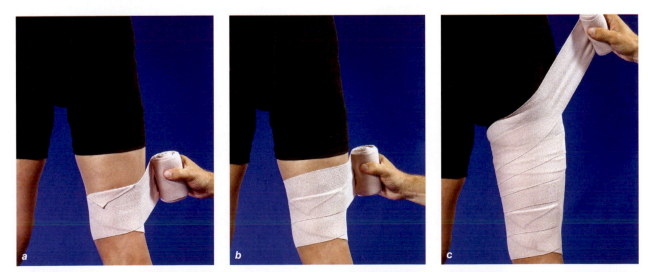

Figure 4.9 Elastic wrap to support a strain of the hamstrings muscles. First, determine if the strain is to the medial or lateral hamstrings. If the medial hamstrings are involved, *(a)* begin by pulling the muscle toward the midline of the posterior thigh, and *(b)* then continue in a circular pattern from the distal to proximal thigh. *(c-d)* Because the hamstrings muscles attach deep beneath the buttock, the wrap will probably be more effective if applied in combination with a hip spica. *(continued)*

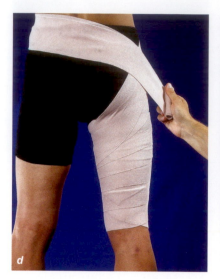
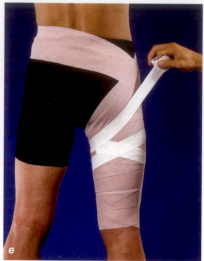
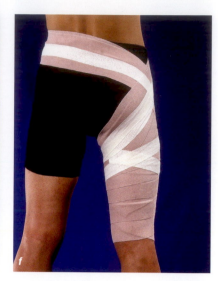

Figure 4.9   *(continued)*   *(e-f)* Trace the wrap with elastic tape.

 Video 4.4 demonstrates testing to determine if a strain involves the medial or lateral hamstring muscles and the application of a figure-eight (spica) elastic wrap traced with elastic tape to support these muscles.

Thigh Exercises

The hamstrings muscles cross the hip and the knee, acting on both joints. Therefore, supplement the stretching and strengthening exercises for hip extensors with those described for knee flexors in chapter 3. Similarly, because the rectus femoris of the quadriceps group crosses both the knee and hip, include the exercises for knee extensors and hip flexors in the patient's regimen.

HIP AND THIGH CONTUSIONS

Hip and thigh contusions involve the **iliac crest** (hip pointer) or quadriceps muscles of the anterior thigh.

Iliac Crest Contusion (Hip Pointer)

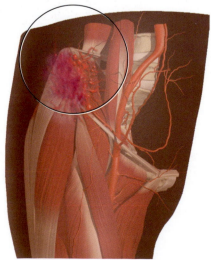

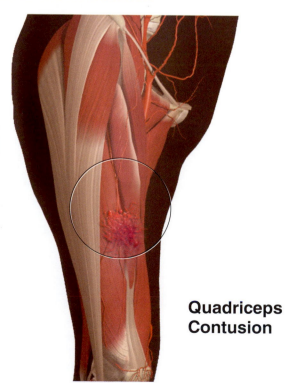

Quadriceps Contusion

Image courtesy of Primal Pictures

Image courtesy of Primal Pictures

Iliac crest injuries, although painful, are not serious. Quadriceps contusions require your special attention because they can create a condition known as **myositis ossificans**, which is the calcification of the **hematoma** caused by a quadriceps bruise.

Hip and Thigh Padding

Use elastic wraps and tape to secure protective pads over the iliac crest or anterior thigh. Figure 4.10 illustrates two ways to position a protective pad over the iliac crest—first with an elastic wrap and then with an elastic wrap and tape hip spica. Figure 4.11 demonstrates how elastic wrap and tape hold a protective pad over the quadriceps.

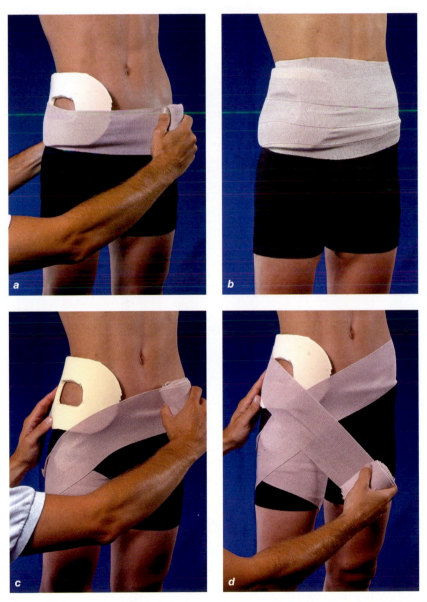

Figure 4.10 An elastic wrap to secure a protective pad over the iliac crest. *(a-b)* Position a pad over the contused iliac crest (hip pointer) and hold it in place with an elastic wrap. *(c-e)* Use a hip spica to provide additional support to the area and to hold the pad in position. *(continued)*

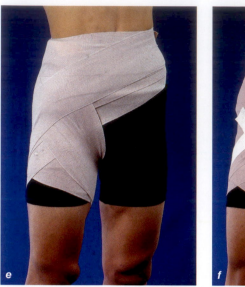
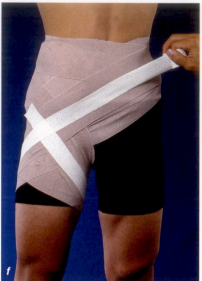
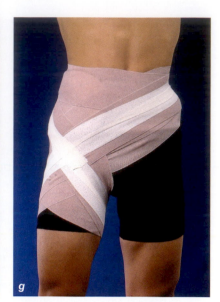

Figure 4.10 *(continued)* *(f-g)* Trace the wrap with elastic tape.

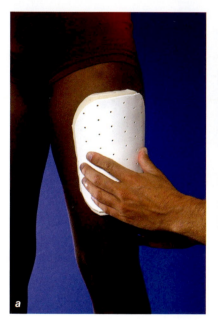
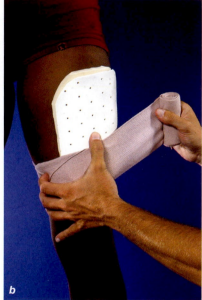
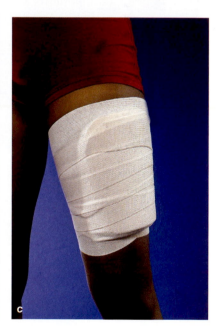

Figure 4.11 *(a-c)* An elastic wrap to secure a protective pad over the quadriceps muscles.

Hip and Thigh Contusion Exercises

The patient should exercise to maintain normal strength and range of motion while hip and thigh contusions heal. Prescribe the stretching and strengthening exercises for both the quadriceps (chapter 3) and hip. Experienced clinicians should monitor serious thigh contusions for the onset of myositis ossificans.

 Visit the web resource for checklists and video clips related to topics discussed in this chapter.

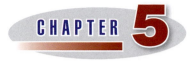
The Shoulder and Arm

The bones of the shoulder girdle include the clavicle, scapula, and humerus. The proximal clavicle and sternum form the sternoclavicular joint, which is the only articulation of the upper extremity with the trunk. The anterior sternoclavicular, posterior sternoclavicular, costoclavicular, and interclavicular ligaments stabilize the joint. The distal clavicle and the acromion process of the scapula create the acromioclavicular joint, an articulation reinforced by the coracoclavicular and acromioclavicular ligaments.

The glenoid cavity of the scapula and the head of the humerus form the shoulder, also known as the glenohumeral joint. The glenoid labrum, the glenohumeral ligaments, and the joint capsule reinforce this shallow, unstable ball-and-socket articulation.

The contraction of the pectoralis major (sternal portion), latissimus dorsi, and teres major muscles causes adduction. The action of the subscapularis and pectoralis major muscles precipitates internal rotation, and the SIT muscles of the rotator cuff—the supraspinatus, infraspinatus, and teres minor—induce external rotation.

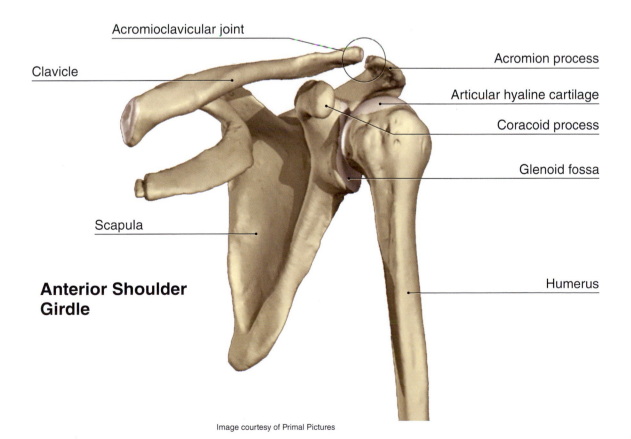

Acromioclavicular joint

Clavicle

Acromion process

Articular hyaline cartilage

Coracoid process

Glenoid fossa

Scapula

Humerus

Anterior Shoulder Girdle

Image courtesy of Primal Pictures

Posterior Shoulder Girdle

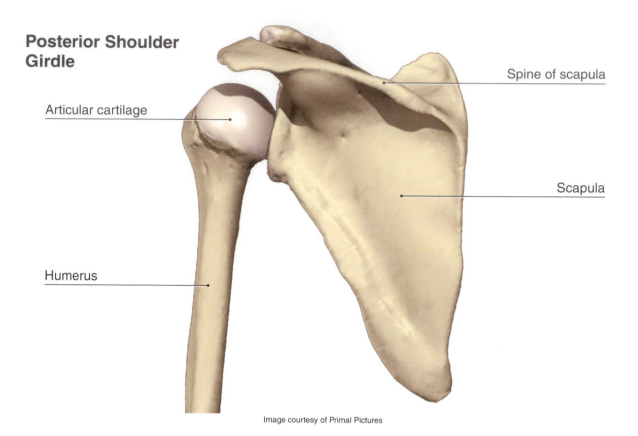

Articular cartilage

Humerus

Spine of scapula

Scapula

Image courtesy of Primal Pictures

Shoulder Complex Ligaments

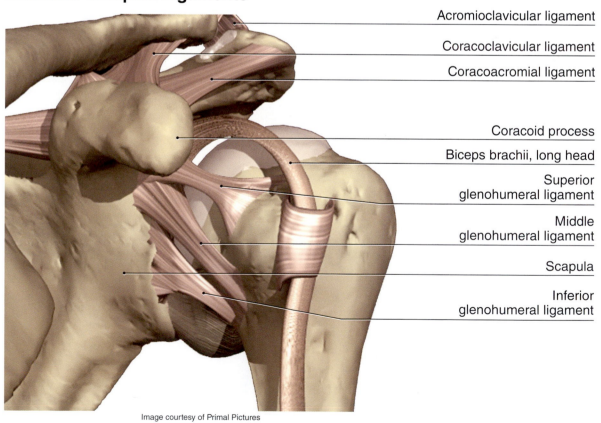

Acromioclavicular ligament

Coracoclavicular ligament

Coracoacromial ligament

Coracoid process

Biceps brachii, long head

Superior
glenohumeral ligament

Middle
glenohumeral ligament

Scapula

Inferior
glenohumeral ligament

Image courtesy of Primal Pictures

The pectoralis major (clavicular portion) and the anterior deltoid produce flexion. Extension results from the latissimus dorsi, teres major, and pectoralis major (sternal portion). Abduction occurs with the deltoid and the **rotator cuff**, whose muscles include the subscapularis, supraspinatus, infraspinatus, and teres minor (figure 5.1).

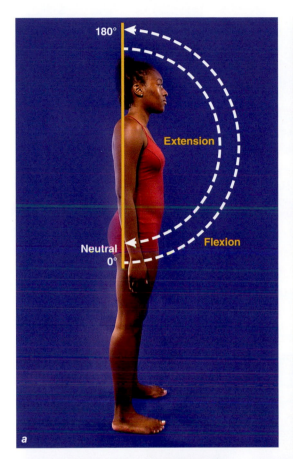

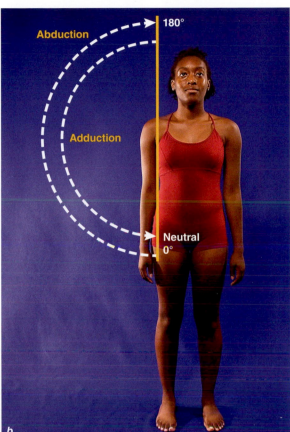

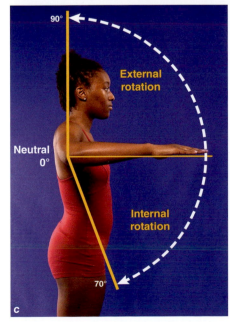

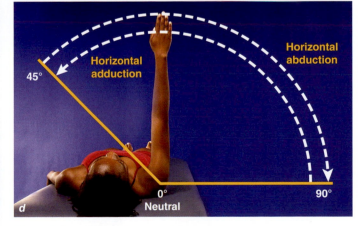

Figure 5.1   *(a)* Shoulder (glenohumeral) flexion and extension ranges of motion; *(b)* shoulder abduction and adduction ranges of motion; *(c)* shoulder internal and external rotation ranges of motion; *(d)* shoulder horizontal adduction and abduction ranges of motion.   *(continued)*

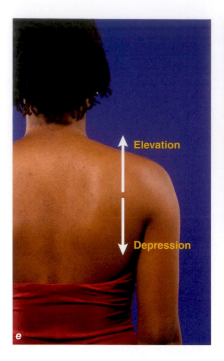

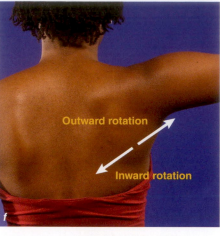

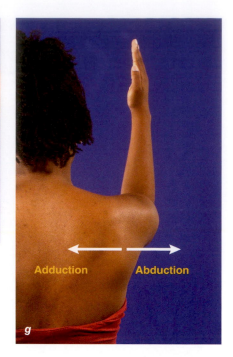

Figure 5.1 *(continued)* Scapular ranges of motion include *(e)* scapular elevation and depression; *(f)* outward and inward rotation; and *(g)* abduction and adduction.

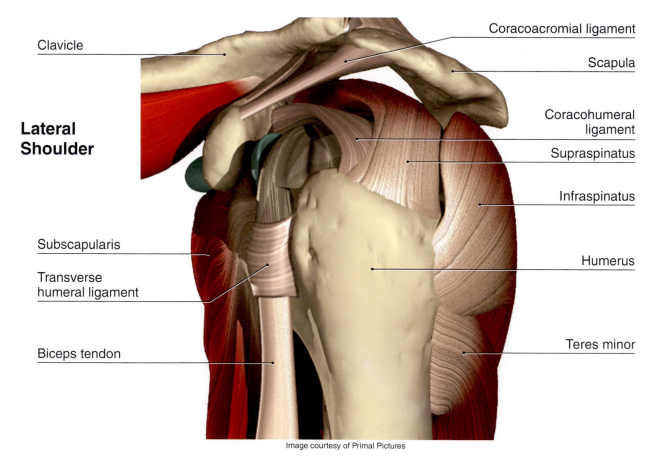

Lateral Shoulder

Clavicle

Coracoacromial ligament

Scapula

Coracohumeral ligament

Supraspinatus

Infraspinatus

Subscapularis

Transverse humeral ligament

Humerus

Biceps tendon

Teres minor

Image courtesy of Primal Pictures

Horizontal flexion occurs with the combination of the coracobrachialis, pectoralis major, and deltoid (anterior portion), and horizontal extension depends on the infraspinatus, teres minor, and deltoid (posterior portion).

The movement of the glenohumeral joint occurs in conjunction with the movement of the scapula. The range of the scapula includes abduction (pectoralis minor and serratus anterior muscles) and adduction (rhomboid muscles), outward rotation (serratus anterior and trapezius muscles) and inward rotation (pectoralis minor and rhomboid muscles), as well as elevation (levator scapulae) and depression (pectoralis minor muscle).

Key Shoulder and Arm Palpation Landmarks

Anterior

▶ Deltoid muscle

▶ Pectoralis major muscle

▶ Clavicle

Posterior

▶ Scapula

Superior

▶ Acromioclavicular joint

Surface Anatomy

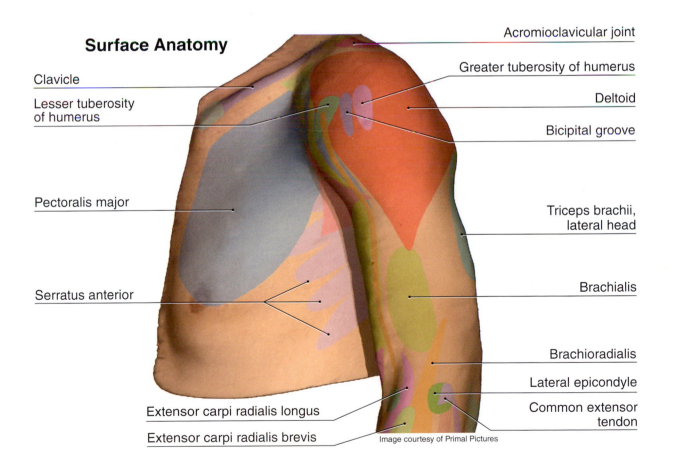

Clavicle

Lesser tuberosity of humerus

Pectoralis major

Serratus anterior

Extensor carpi radialis longus

Extensor carpi radialis brevis

Acromioclavicular joint

Greater tuberosity of humerus

Deltoid

Bicipital groove

Triceps brachii, lateral head

Brachialis

Brachioradialis

Lateral epicondyle

Common extensor tendon

Image courtesy of Primal Pictures

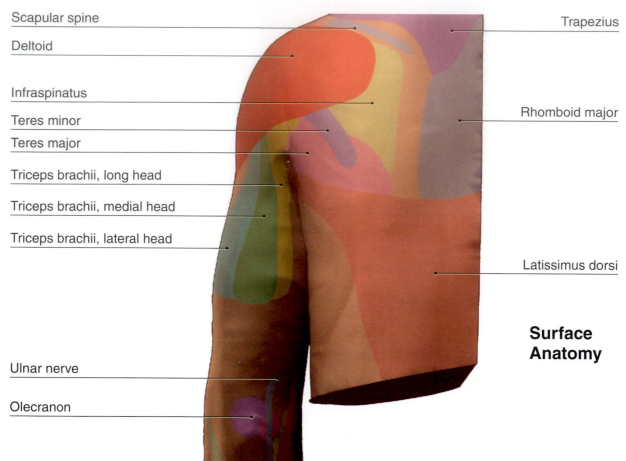

Scapular spine

Deltoid

Infraspinatus

Teres minor

Teres major

Triceps brachii, long head

Triceps brachii, medial head

Triceps brachii, lateral head

Ulnar nerve

Olecranon

Trapezius

Rhomboid major

Latissimus dorsi

**Surface
Anatomy**

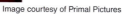
Image courtesy of Primal Pictures

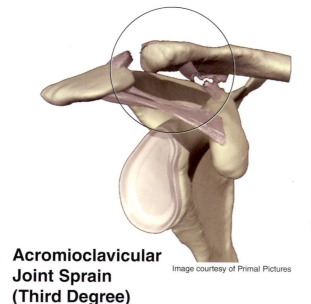

**Acromioclavicular
Joint Sprain
(Third Degree)**

Image courtesy of Primal Pictures

ACROMIOCLAVICULAR
JOINT SPRAINS

Athletes suffer an **acromioclavicular joint sprain** (known colloquially as a separated shoulder) when they fall on the hand, elbow, or the shoulder itself. Clinicians categorize the sprains as first- to third-degree injuries. The first degree describes a minor tear of the acromioclavicular ligament, and the third degree refers to a complete rupture of both the acromioclavicular and coracoclavicular ligaments. In the latter case, the shoulder drops and the clavicle protrudes against the skin of the superior shoulder.

Acromioclavicular Joint Taping

Begin taping an acromioclavicular joint sprain by placing anchor strips around the arm, over the top of the shoulder, and on the chest and back (figure 5.2). Make certain that when taping the shoulder or chest you protect the nipple with gauze or a bandage. Continue taping with successive strips from the arm anchor to the shoulder anchor and from the chest anchor to the back anchor.

 Video 5.1 demonstrates taping and padding procedures to protect a sprained acromioclavicular joint.

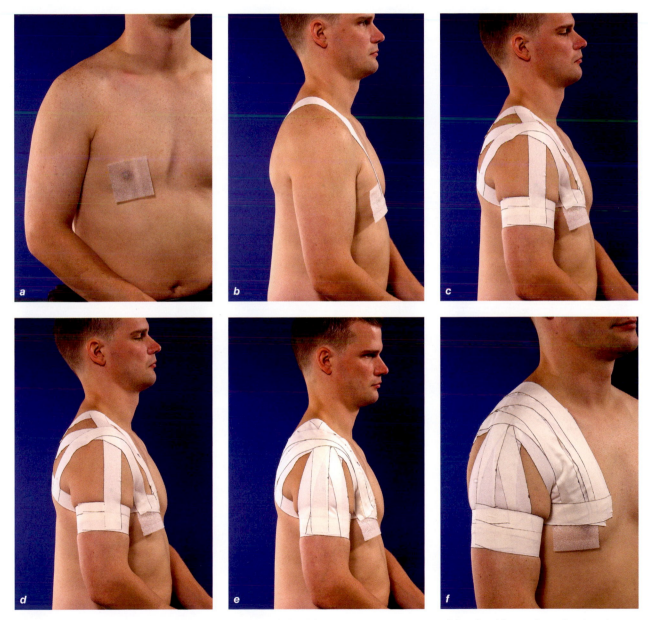

Figure 5.2   Acromioclavicular joint sprain (separated shoulder) taping. *(a)* Any taping of the shoulder or chest that has the potential to cover the nipple should begin with the application of protective dressing. *(b)* Apply anchor strips to the superior, anterior, and posterior aspects of the shoulder as well as *(c)* to the proximal arm. *(d-f)* Apply strips from the arm anchor to the superior shoulder anchor and from the anterior to posterior anchors in an overlapping fashion so that the crossing point of the tape is over the acromioclavicular joint.

You may supplement or replace this procedure by using a protective pad over the injured acromioclavicular joint. Figure 5.3 illustrates the technique for making a protective pad from orthoplast and how to secure the pad with an elastic-wrap shoulder spica. You can use this technique for making a custom-fitted protective pad to protect other injuries, such as contusions of the quadriceps, iliac crest, and a blocker's exostosis.

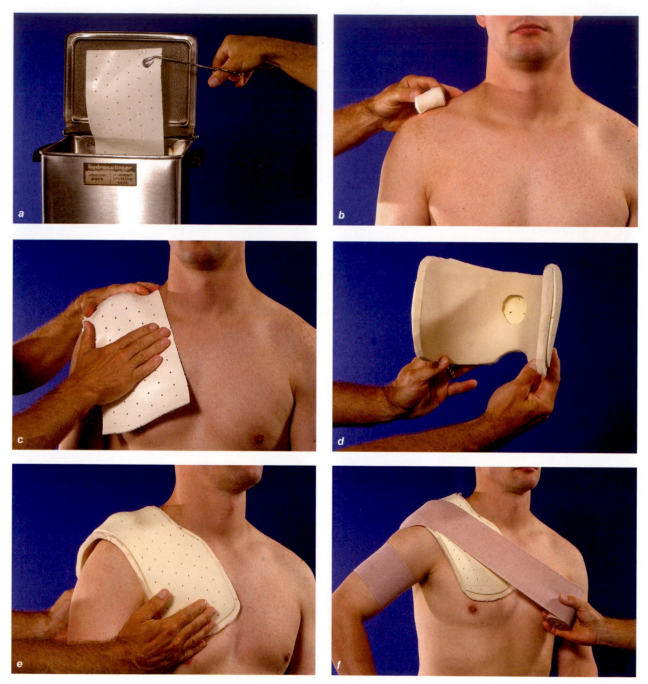

Figure 5.3   *(a-e)* Produce a protective pad from orthoplast and *(f-i)* secure the pad in place with an elastic-wrap shoulder spica.   *(continued)*

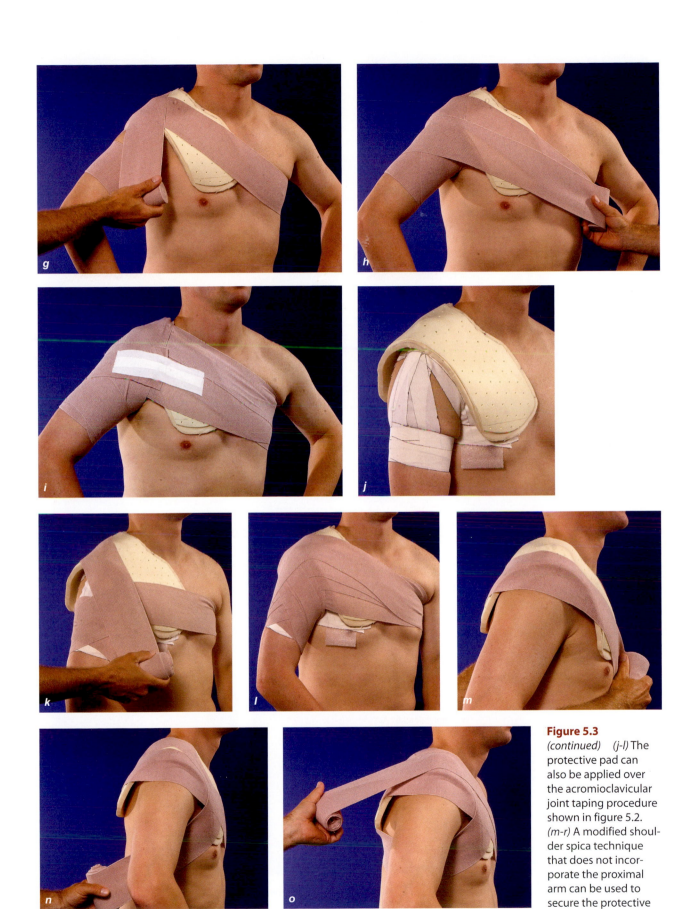

Figure 5.3
(continued) *(j-l)* The protective pad can also be applied over the acromioclavicular joint taping procedure shown in figure 5.2. *(m-r)* A modified shoulder spica technique that does not incorporate the proximal arm can be used to secure the protective pad. *(continued)*

111

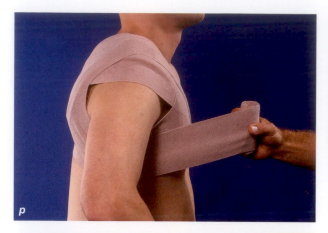

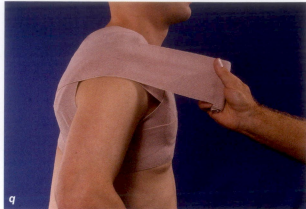

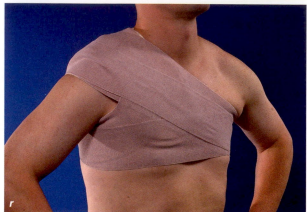

Figure 5.3 *(continued)*

McConnell Taping for Acromioclavicular Joint Sprains

You can use the same kind of tape used for McConnell taping of the patella (see figure 3.16) for acromioclavicular joint sprains. This taping procedure can be left in place for an extended period and will help "reapproximate" the acromioclavicular joint (figure 5.4).

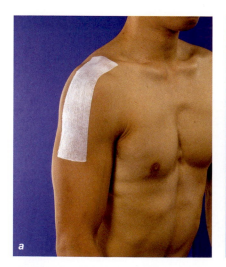

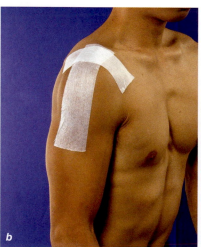

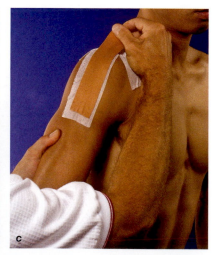

Figure 5.4 McConnell taping for an acromioclavicular joint sprain. Use underwrap stretch and strapping tape as with the McConnell taping for patellofemoral joint pain. *(a)* Apply the first underwrap strip vertically from the deltoid tuberosity past the acromioclavicular joint by 3/4 to 1-1/4 inches (2-3 cm). *(b)* Apply the second strip from the coracoid process to the spine of the scapula. *(c)* Apply the first strapping tape strip vertically over the underwrap strip while approximating the acromioclavicular joint. *(continued)*

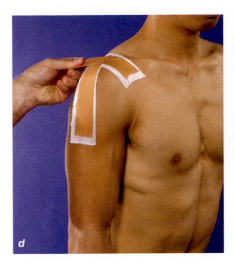

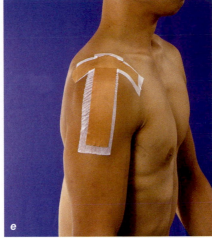

Figure 5.4 *(continued)* *(d)* Apply the second strip of strapping tape anterior to posterior. *(e)* The point of the crossing strips should center over the acromioclavicular joint. An additional layer of strapping tape strips may be necessary to provide ample support.

Shoulder Exercises

Most sports, especially those that require overhead arm motion, rely on adequate strength and flexibility of the shoulder. Construct a simple T-bar for exercises to stretch the shoulder (figure 5.5). Be certain that the exercise regimen addresses the full range of motion of the shoulder.

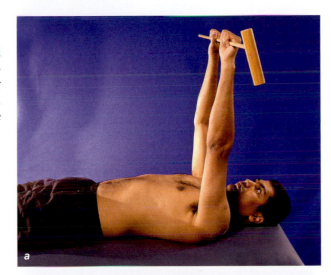

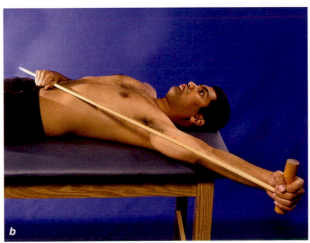

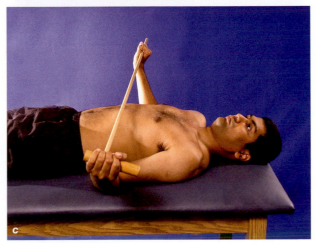

Figure 5.5 A simple T-bar to stretch the shoulder muscles through *(a)* flexion, *(b)* abduction, and *(c)* external rotation.

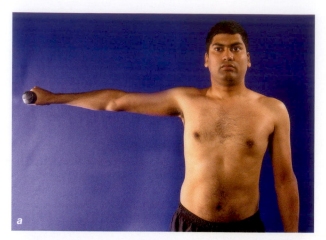

Strengthening exercises employ dumbbells, elastic bands, or a combination of both devices. Figure 5.6 illustrates how a hand-held weight provides resistance through each of the motions of the shoulder. Elastic bands can supply similar resistance while also allowing for exercise that traces functional movement patterns (figure 5.7).

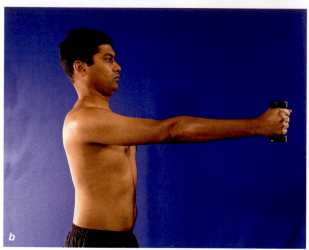

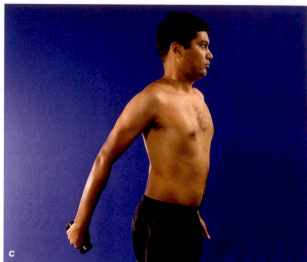

Figure 5.6   A hand-held weight to strengthen the shoulder *(a)* abductor, *(b)* flexor, and *(c)* extensor muscles. Normally, these motions should not exceed the horizontal positions seen in *(a)* and *(b)*.

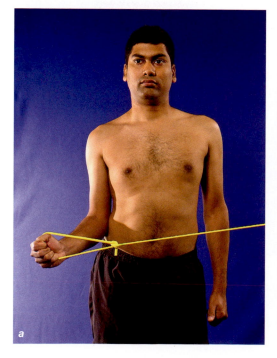

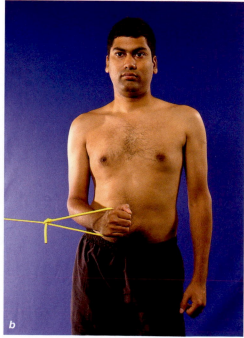

Figure 5.7   Elastic bands are effective for strengthening the shoulder *(a)* external and *(b)* internal rotator muscles.

GLENOHUMERAL SPRAINS

Sprains, **subluxations**, and **dislocations**, all common injuries of the glenohumeral joint, cause the shoulder to be chronically unstable. The patient often requires surgery to repair the damage. Although congenital factors may contribute to the injuries, sprains or dislocations usually occur when the patient applies an external force to the arm. Shoulder abduction and external rotation are the common mechanisms of injury for anterior dislocation.

Shoulder Sprain or Instability Taping

Your taping procedure should prevent excessive abduction and external rotation. An elastic-wrap shoulder spica, traced with elastic tape, limits these motions (figure 5.8). Have the patient internally rotate the shoulder and begin taping by encircling the arm and crossing over the anterior chest; this action pulls the shoulder into internal rotation and limits external rotation. The amount of mobility that the patient requires will dictate the degree of limitation that you provide.

 Video 5.2 demonstrates the application of a figure-eight shoulder (spica) with elastic wrap to support a sprained shoulder.

In addition to elastic wraps, shoulder braces restrict abduction and external rotation (figure 5.9). You can adjust their restriction from a minimal to a substantial amount.

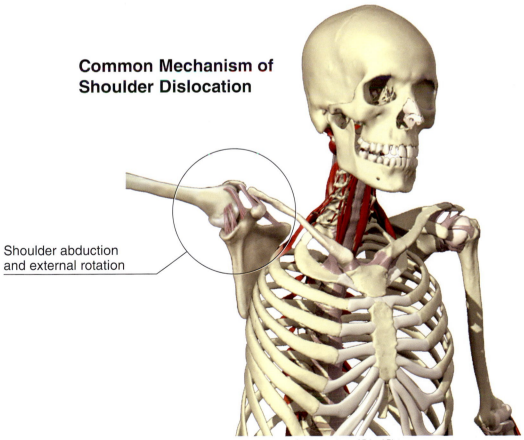

Common Mechanism of Shoulder Dislocation

Shoulder abduction and external rotation

Image courtesy of Primal Pictures

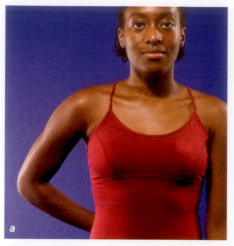
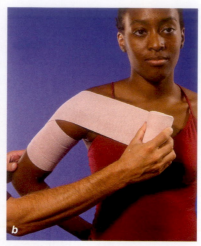

Figure 5.8 An elastic-wrap shoulder spica with tape to support the unstable shoulder. *(a)* The procedure begins by having the patient place the shoulder in an internally rotated position with the hand on the hip. *(b)* Start the wrap on the arm and pull medially across the anterior chest. *(c-e)* The wrap continues around the arm and again proceeds around the chest. *(f-h)* Use elastic tape to trace the elastic wrap.

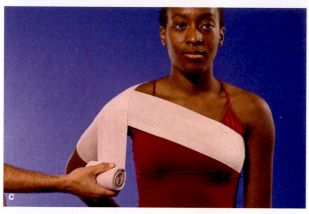
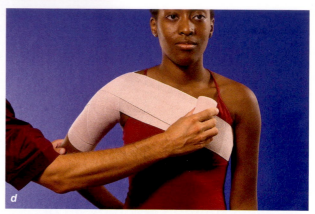

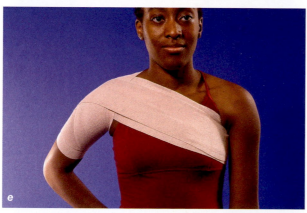
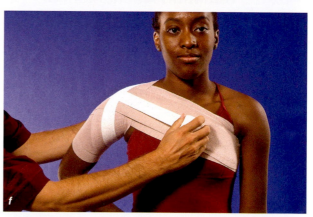

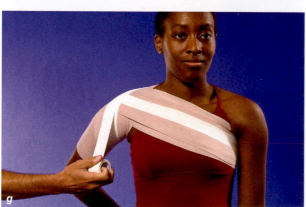
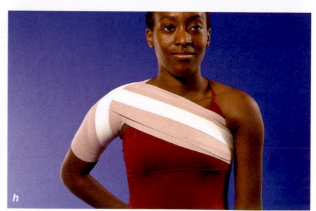

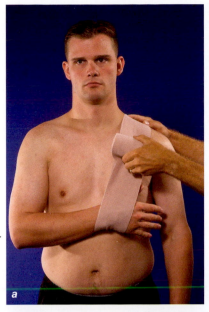

a

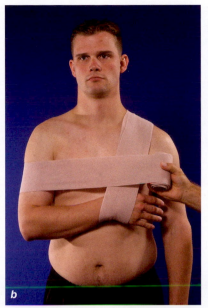

b

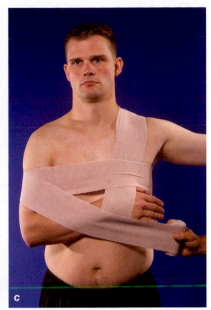

c

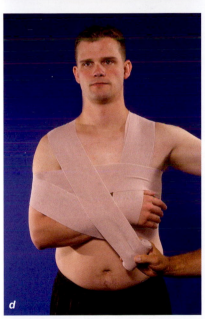

d

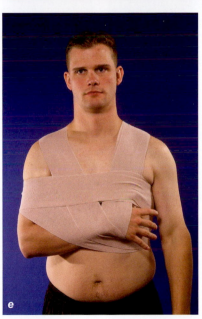

e

Figure 5.9 *(a-e)* An elastic wrap can immobilize an acutely injured shoulder. *(f-g)* A commercially produced brace can limit shoulder abduction and external rotation. Control the degree of abduction through the adjustable straps of the brace.

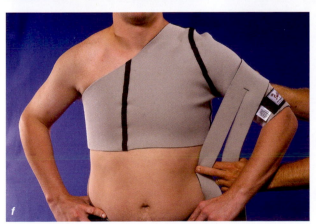

f

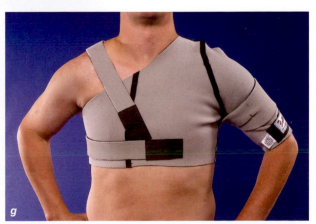

g

Kinesiology tape can be useful when full shoulder motion is required and in the presence of pain due to shoulder hypermobility (anterior or multi-axial), subacromial bursitis, or scapulohumeral dysfunction (figure 5.10). If control of laxity is required, use an athletic taping technique.

 Video 5.3 demonstrates kinesiology taping to provide stability to a shoulder with joint laxity.

Shoulder Sprain or Instability Exercises

Combine the exercises illustrated in figures 5.5 through 5.7 with the shoulder wrapping and bracing procedures. Do not, however, prescribe the stretching exercises that enhance shoulder abduction and external rotation, because, in this case, the exercises would stress an unstable shoulder that is already hypermobile. Have the patient focus on internal-rotation strengthening exercises because they will limit the external rotation of the shoulder.

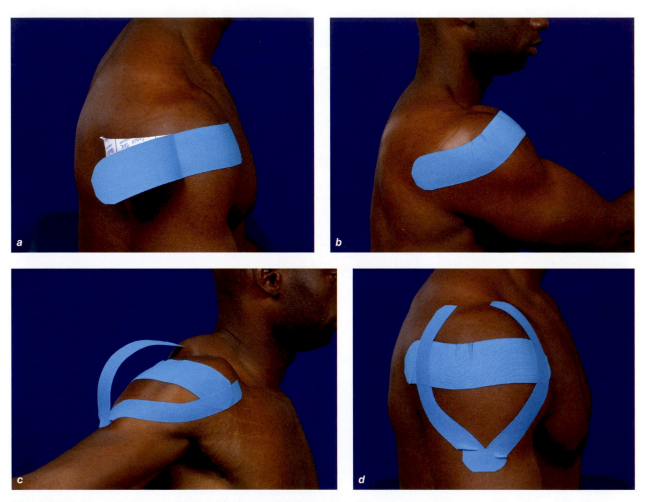

Figure 5.10   Kinesiology taping for shoulder laxity. With the patient sitting, measure and cut tape from the length of the anterior shoulder around the deltoid to the posterior shoulder. Cut edges round. *(a)* Fully retract scapula and start to tape, then apply tension from the anterior shoulder to middle deltoid, *(b)* then horizontally adduct and flex the shoulder to fix the posterior end of the tape without tension. For an optional deltoid piece, cut a strip longer than the length from the AC to the mid-deltoid insertion and cut a Y. *(c)* Start at the mid-deltoid, horizontally abduct the shoulder and place the anterior deltoid piece without tension, and end medial to the AC joint. Place shoulder in horizontal adduction and place the posterior deltoid piece, ending posterior to the AC joint. The final result is shown in *d*.

ARM CONTUSIONS

Athletes often suffer arm contusions, especially when playing football or other contact sports. Arm contusions, like those of the thigh, may develop myositis ossificans, an injury termed blocker's **exostosis**.

Arm Contusion Taping

Protect the arm from repeated trauma by securing a protective pad to the area. Figure 5.11 illustrates how to use elastic tape when applying a protective pad to the lateral aspect of the arm.

Arm Contusion Exercises

The exercises illustrated in figures 5.5 through 5.7 and those for the elbow in chapter 6 will help the injured patient maintain normal strength and flexibility. An experienced clinician should monitor the injury for exostosis in the soft tissue of the arm and prescribe rest if this condition develops.

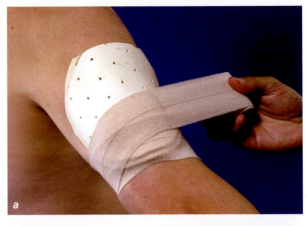

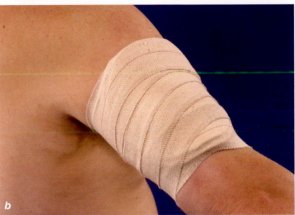

Figure 5.11 *(a-b)* Elastic tape to secure a protective pad to the arm.

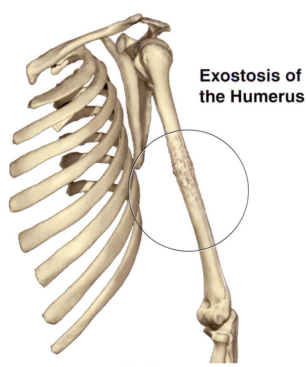

Exostosis of the Humerus

Image courtesy of Primal Pictures

 Visit the web resource for checklists and video clips related to topics discussed in this chapter.

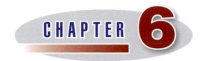

The Elbow and Forearm

The joining of the distal humerus with the proximal ulna forms the elbow. The medial collateral ligament, called the ulnar, and lateral collateral ligament, referred to as the radial, limit valgus and varus displacement, respectively.

Anterior Elbow

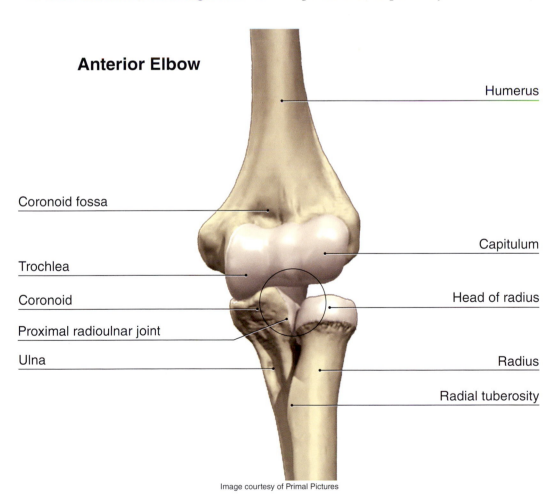

Coronoid fossa

Trochlea

Coronoid

Proximal radioulnar joint

Ulna

Humerus

Capitulum

Head of radius

Radius

Radial tuberosity

Image courtesy of Primal Pictures

Posterior Elbow

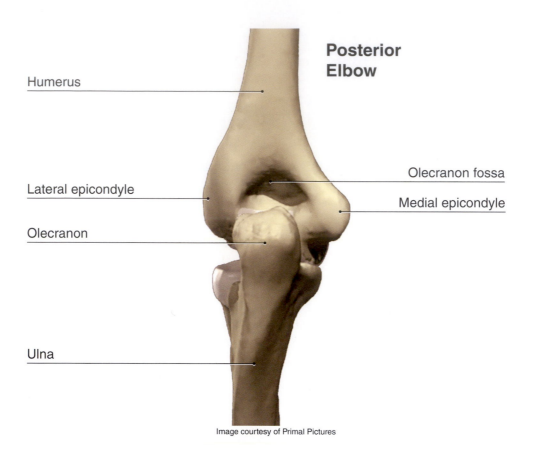

Humerus

Lateral epicondyle

Olecranon

Ulna

Olecranon fossa

Medial epicondyle

Image courtesy of Primal Pictures

Elbow Joint Ligaments

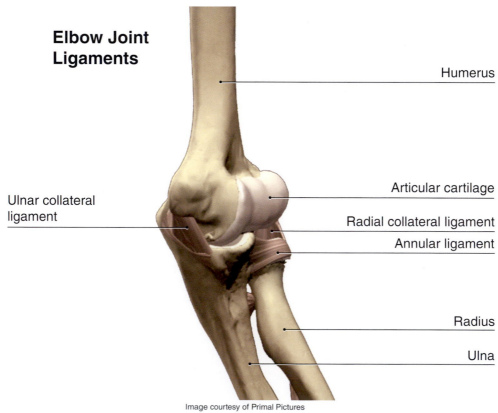

Ulnar collateral ligament

Humerus

Articular cartilage

Radial collateral ligament

Annular ligament

Radius

Ulna

Image courtesy of Primal Pictures

Lateral Shoulder and Arm

Subacromial bursa

Infraspinatus

Teres minor

Humerus

Pectoralis minor

Triceps brachii, long head

Biceps brachii, long head

Triceps brachii, lateral head

Brachialis

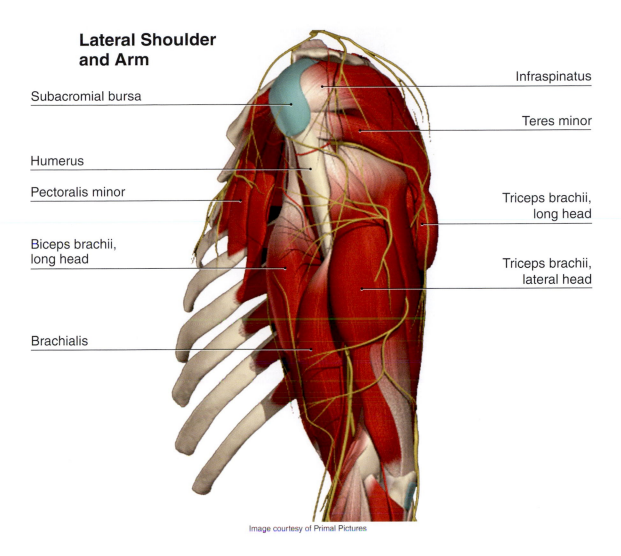

Image courtesy of Primal Pictures

The hinge of the elbow permits flexion and extension (figure 6.1a). Flexion occurs through the action of the anterior muscles of the arm, which include the biceps brachii and brachialis. The three heads of the triceps brachii comprise the posterior muscles and produce elbow extension.

The radius and ulna of the forearm create three joints: the proximal radioulnar, the distal radioulnar, and the articulation along the shafts of both bones. The fibers of the annular ligament stabilize the proximal radioulnar joint. The interosseous membrane joins the shafts of the radius and ulna, and an articular capsule supports the distal radioulnar joint. Pronation and supination describe the potential movements of the forearm (figure 6.1b). The pronator teres and pronator quadratus muscles cause pronation, and the supinator muscle produces supination.

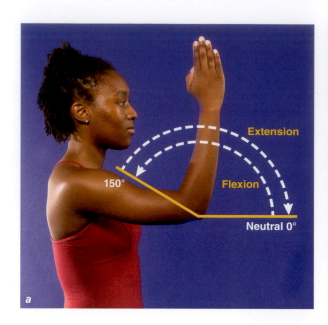
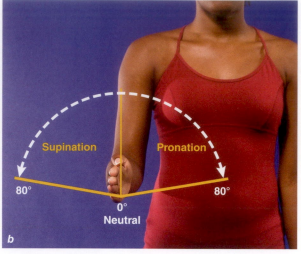

Figure 6.1 *(a)* Elbow flexion and extension ranges of motion. *(b)* Forearm pronation and supination ranges of motion.

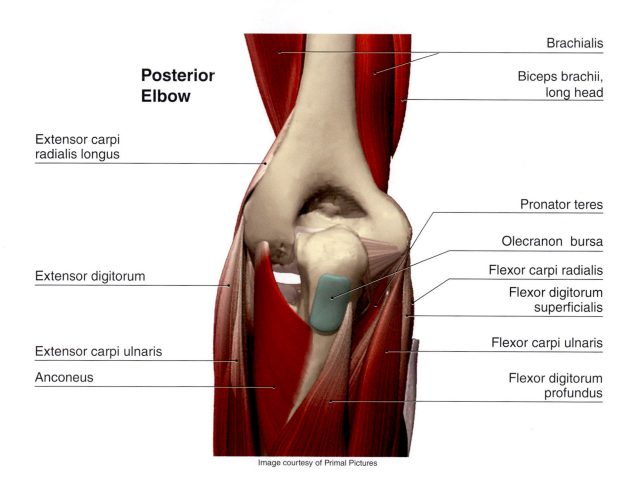

Posterior Elbow

Brachialis

Biceps brachii, long head

Extensor carpi radialis longus

Pronator teres

Olecranon bursa

Flexor carpi radialis

Extensor digitorum

Flexor digitorum superficialis

Flexor carpi ulnaris

Extensor carpi ulnaris

Anconeus

Flexor digitorum profundus

Image courtesy of Primal Pictures

Key Elbow and Forearm Palpation Landmarks

Anterior

► Cubital fossa
► Biceps tendon

Medial

► Ulnar nerve
► Wrist flexor-pronator group
► Medial epicondyle
► Medial collateral ligament
► Ulna

Lateral

► Wrist extensor-supinator muscle group
► Lateral epicondyle
► Lateral collateral ligament
► Radius

Posterior

► Olecranon process
► Olecranon bursa
► Triceps muscle

ELBOW SPRAINS

Similar to knee injuries, elbow sprains occur when valgus or varus forces damage the medial or lateral collateral ligaments, respectively. Sports that depend on the patient's overarm throwing ability will impart chronic stress to the medial compartment of the elbow and injure the medial collateral ligament.

Elbow Sprain Taping

Medial and lateral instabilities can be difficult injuries to support, and taping the elbow is unlikely to help the patient who suffers from chronic stress to the medial collateral ligament. Figure 6.2, however, illustrates a collateral ligament taping procedure that you may find valuable for some cases. The procedure is remarkably similar to taping the collateral ligaments of the knee (see chapter 3).

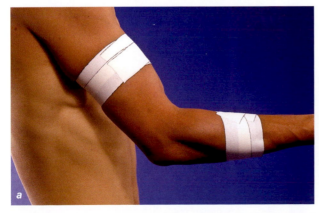
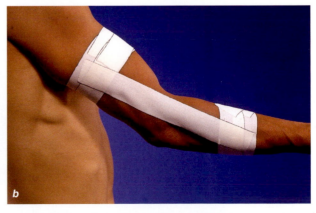

Figure 6.2   Elbow collateral ligament taping for instability of the lateral collateral ligament. *(a)* The procedure begins with proximal and distal anchor strips. *(b-d)* Place strips over the lateral collateral ligament in an X fashion.   *(continued)*

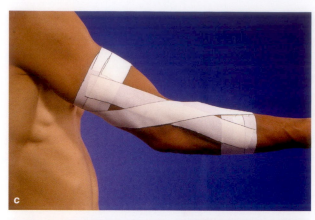

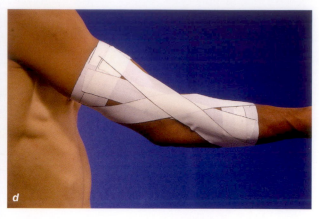

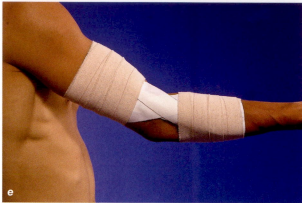

Figure 6.2 *(continued)*   (e) Secure the tape with proximal and distal anchors using elastic tape that encloses all but the elbow joint itself.

 Video 6.1 demonstrates taping for instability resulting from an injury to the medial or lateral collateral ligaments of the elbow.

Elbow Exercises

Stretch the elbow flexor and extensor muscles with the assistance of the contralateral extremity (figure 6.3).

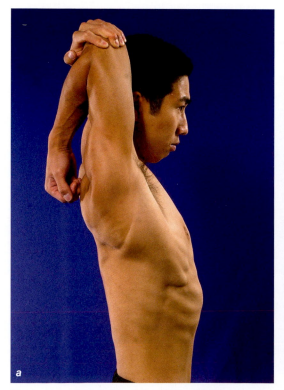

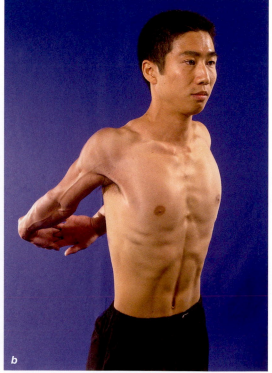

Figure 6.3   Stretching of the elbow *(a)* extensor and *(b)* flexor muscles with the contralateral extremity.

Strengthening exercises should work the muscles that produce elbow flexion and extension, forearm pronation and supination, and wrist flexion and extension. We recommend a combination of hand-held weights and elastic bands, as figure 6.4 illustrates. Chapter 7 will discuss exercises for the wrist.

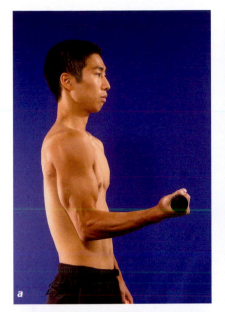

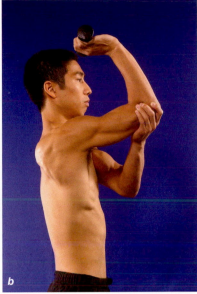

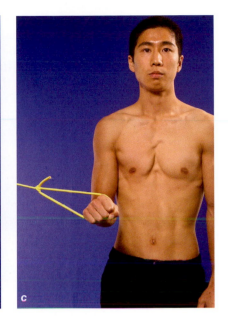

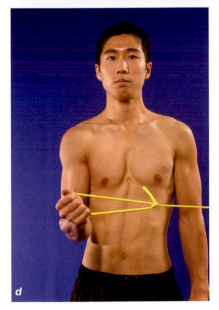

Figure 6.4 Strengthening exercises for the elbow (a) flexor and (b) extensor muscles with a hand-held weight. Elastic bands will strengthen the forearm (c) pronator and (d) supinator muscles.

ELBOW HYPEREXTENSION

Self-inflicted or external forces can extend the elbow beyond its normal anatomical limit; the motion produces a hyperextension injury that damages the ulna or humerus where it articulates during extension. The soft-tissue structures on the anterior aspect of the elbow could also suffer trauma. In severe cases, hyperextension will fracture or dislocate the elbow.

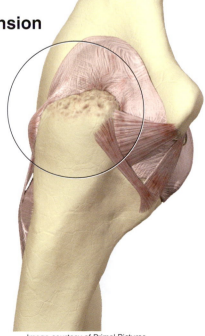

Elbow Hyperextension Injury

Image courtesy of Primal Pictures

Elbow Hyperextension Taping

Elbow and knee hyperextension share a similar taping procedure (see chapter 3). Determine the degree of extension that produces discomfort and slightly flex the joint for the duration of the taping. Place anchor strips around the arm and forearm (figure 6.5). To prevent slippage, we recommend that you apply the anchors directly to the skin. You may also find it advantageous to secure the proximal anchor above the belly of the biceps. Tape successive, interlocking strips over the anterior aspect of the elbow. Elastic tape works well when supporting hyperextension injuries. If necessary, complete the taping procedure by enclosing the elbow with elastic tape or wrap.

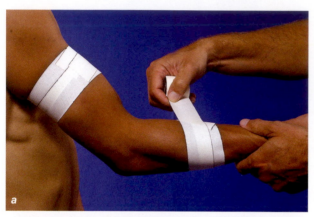

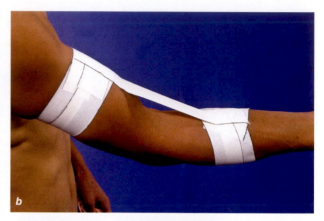

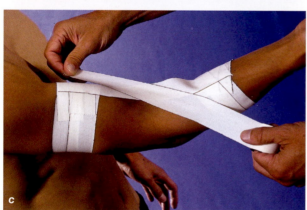

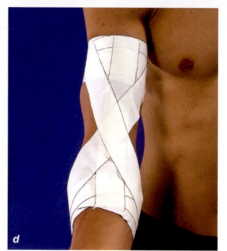

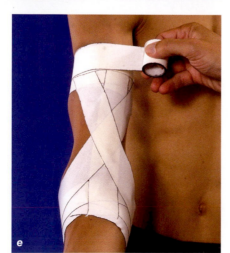

Figure 6.5 Elbow hyperextension taping procedure. *(a)* Begin the procedure on a shaved arm and apply proximal and distal anchor strips. *(b-d)* Form an X with three strips of tape over the anterior aspect of the elbow. *(e)* Apply proximal and distal anchor strips to secure the tape.   *(continued)*

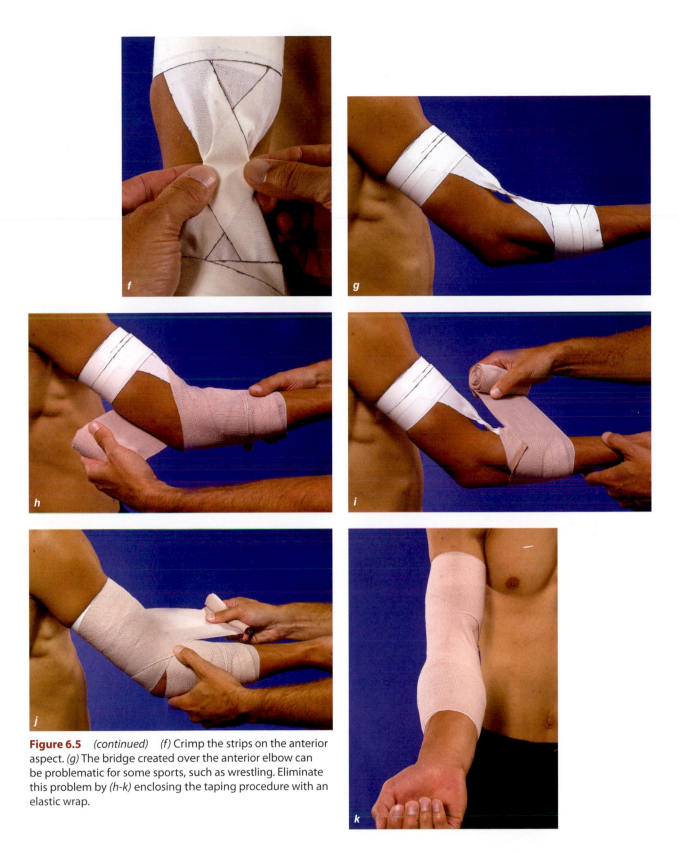

Figure 6.5 *(continued)* *(f)* Crimp the strips on the anterior aspect. *(g)* The bridge created over the anterior elbow can be problematic for some sports, such as wrestling. Eliminate this problem by *(h-k)* enclosing the taping procedure with an elastic wrap.

▶ Video 6.2 demonstrates a taping procedure to limit extension in the hyperextended elbow.

Kinesiology taping is an alternative technique when full elbow motion and extension is necessary (figure 6.6). However, it is not as supportive as the athletic taping technique.

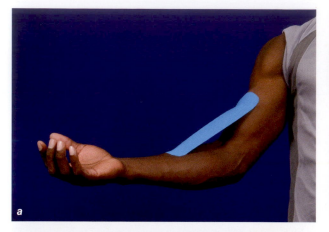

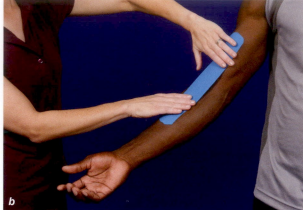

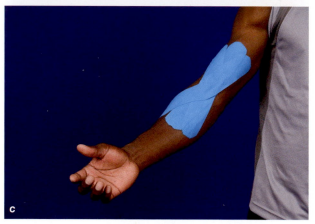

Figure 6.6   Kinesiology taping for elbow hyperextension laxity. With the patient standing, measure and cut three pieces of tape 12 to 16 inches (30-40 cm) long. Determine the degree of elbow extension to be limited. *(a)* Apply tape with the patient flexing the elbow more than this amount, anchoring the first piece 5 to 6 inches (13-15 cm) superior and inferior to the elbow. *(b)* Have the patient slowly extend the elbow as the tape is secured with maximal tension from both ends toward the cubital fossa. *(c)* A reinforcing application crosses the strips with tension at the cubital fossa, keeping the elbow flexed.

▶ Video 6.3 demonstrates kinesiology taping for elbow hyperextension laxity.

In cases in which maximal stability is desired, a hinged elbow brace can be utilized (figure 6.7*a*). An advantage of the hinged elbow brace is that it not only supports the collateral ligaments but also allows the clinician to adjust the allowable range of motion (figure 6.7*b*).

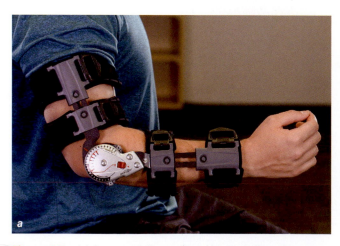

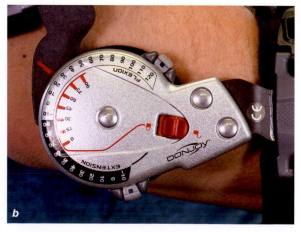

Figure 6.7   *(a)* Commercially produced hinged elbow brace to support collateral ligaments and adjust allowable range of motion. *(b)* Close-up of adjustable range of motion dial on hinged elbow brace.

Hyperextension Exercises

Figure 6.3 details extension and flexion exercises that will restore the normal range of motion of the injured elbow. The strengthening regimen needs to isolate the elbow flexor and extensor muscles (see figure 6.4).

EPICONDYLITIS OF THE HUMERUS

The medial and lateral epicondyles of the humerus attach with several muscles. Muscles originate from the lateral epicondyle for forearm supination and wrist extension. The medial epicondyle joins with muscles for forearm pronation and wrist flexion. Repetitive forearm and wrist motion—such as that required for tennis or throwing—inflames these muscles at their points of origin from the medial or lateral epicondyles. Tennis players commonly suffer from lateral **epicondylitis**, known colloquially as tennis elbow. Athletes who repeatedly use a throwing motion, especially adolescents, frequently experience medial epicondylitis, often called Little Leaguer's elbow.

Epicondylitis Taping

We have found that taping for epicondylitis is not always effective. Some patients experience relief from strips of tape applied to compress the proximal forearm (figure 6.8). Commercially produced braces will also serve this purpose (figure 6.9). In adults, strap taping for medial or lateral epicondylitis can

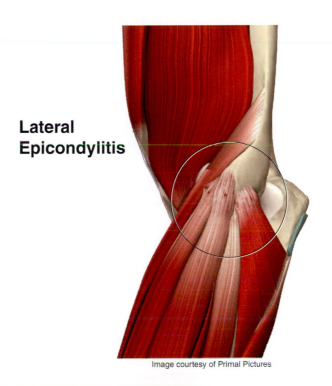

Lateral Epicondylitis

Image courtesy of Primal Pictures

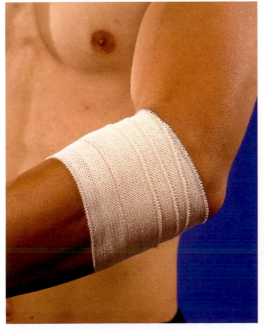

Figure 6.8 The application of tape around the proximal forearm can sometimes alleviate pain associated with lateral epicondylitis (tennis elbow).

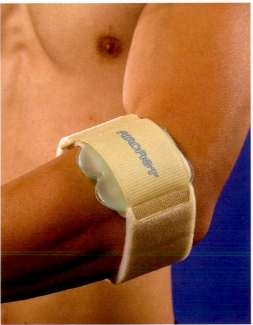

Figure 6.9 A commercially produced brace can also alleviate pain associated with lateral epicondylitis.

be very effective as an alternative to braces, because braces can often be bulky or ill-fitting. Strapping tape can be left on for days. This one technique will help both types of epicondylitis (figure 6.10).

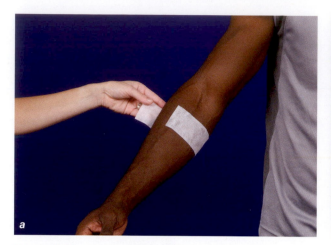 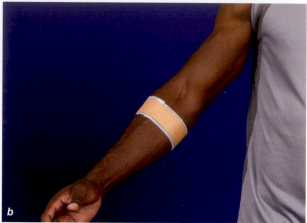

Figure 6.10   Epicondylitis strapping. *(a)* With the patient sitting or standing, apply underwrap approximately 2 inches (5 cm) distal to the elbow and around the circumference of the forearm. Apply strapping tape with some force so that when the patient grips, the pain is decreased at the elbow and felt as tightness under the tape. The final result is shown in *b*.

 Video 6.4 demonstrates epicondylitis strapping.

Exercise caution when treating medial epicondylitis in an adolescent patient. For many adolescents, the strength of the muscles exceeds the tolerance of the immature bone. The throwing mechanism may cause **avulsion** fractures of the medial epicondyle. For this reason, do not tape an adolescent patient so that he or she throws through the discomfort associated with medial epicondylitis.

Epicondylitis Exercises

After the inflammation associated with lateral epicondylitis has resolved, prescribe exercises to enhance the patient's range of motion and strength. The stretching exercises for the elbow and forearm will increase flexibility. For lateral epicondylitis, hyperflex the wrist during complete pronation (figure 6.11). The strengthening techniques should exercise the forearm supinators and wrist extensors (chapter 7). Rest is the best treatment for medial epicondylitis.

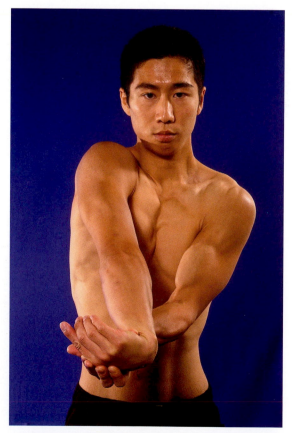

Figure 6.11   Stretching of the extensor-supinator muscles commonly implicated in lateral epicondylitis.

FRACTURES OF THE FOREARM

Fractures of the forearm include isolated ulnar shaft fractures and combined ulnar shaft and radial shaft fractures. Isolated ulnar shaft fractures are also known as "night stick" fractures because the common mechanism of injury is a direct blow to the ulnar shaft. The primary difference between the isolated ulnar shaft fracture and combined ulnar shaft and radial shaft fractures is that the ulnar shaft fracture is considered a stable fracture because the uncompromised radial shaft provides stability to the forearm. In contrast, the combined ulnar shaft and radial shaft fractures are inherently unstable due to the involvement of both bones.

The mechanism of injury for the combined fractures is either from a direct blow of great force or a fall on the outstretched arm. Due to the unstable nature of combined forearm fractures, best outcomes are obtained with surgical fixation of the fractures.

Elbow dislocations are less common than forearm fractures, but there is a high risk of neurovascular injury with dislocations; therefore, it is extremely important that elbow dislocations are immobilized to prevent further injury. The common mechanism of injury for elbow dislocations is falling on the outstretched arm with the elbow fully extended.

Methods for Immobilizing the Fractured Forearm

Immobilization of the fractured forearm can be accomplished with splints or casts such as a sugar tong splint, double sugar tong splint, or ulnar shaft fracture cast. An isolated ulnar shaft fracture is initially splinted, but once the post-traumatic swelling has resolved, it is immobilized with an ulnar shaft fracture cast (figure 6.12). Sugar tong splints (figure 6.13) are used when a stable fracture is present and double sugar tong splints (figure 6.14) are used for unstable fractures and other types of unstable injuries such as elbow dislocations. Similar to double sugar tong splints, long arm casts (figure 6.15) immobilize the wrist, forearm, and elbow, which makes them ideal for immobilizing unstable forearm fractures that do not require surgical fixation.

Isolated Ulnar Shaft Fracture

Combined Ulnar Shaft and Radial Shaft Fractures

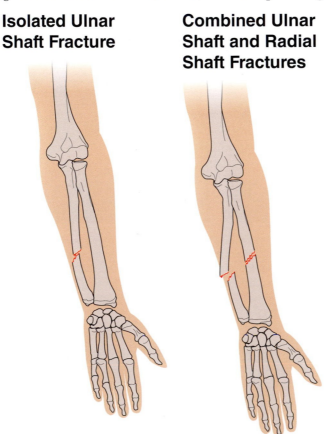

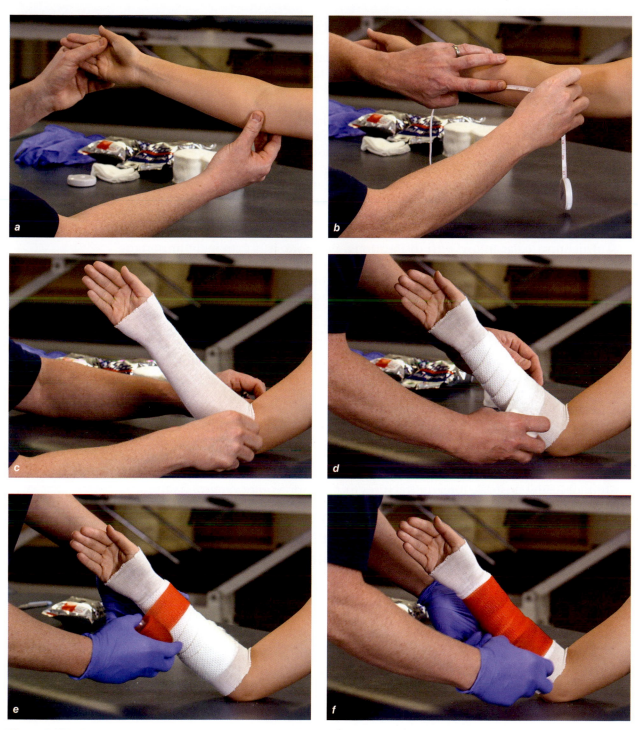

Figure 6.12 Casting procedure for an isolated ulnar shaft fracture. *(a)* Position the forearm in 0° of pronation. *(b)* Measure 2 inches (5 cm) beyond the antecubital fossa and 2 inches (5 cm) beyond the proximal wrist crease to determine the amount of stockinette needed. *(c)* Apply the stockinette. *(d)* Beginning at the proximal wrist crease, roll the cast padding circumferentially from distal to proximal, overlapping by 50% to end just below antecubital fossa. *(e)* Starting 2 to 3 finger widths above the proximal wrist crease, begin applying the fiberglass from distal to proximal, overlapping the previous layer by 50%. *(f)* End the fiberglass 2 to 3 finger widths below the antecubital fossa.   *(continued)*

 Video 6.5 demonstrates the casting procedure for an isolated ulnar shaft fracture.

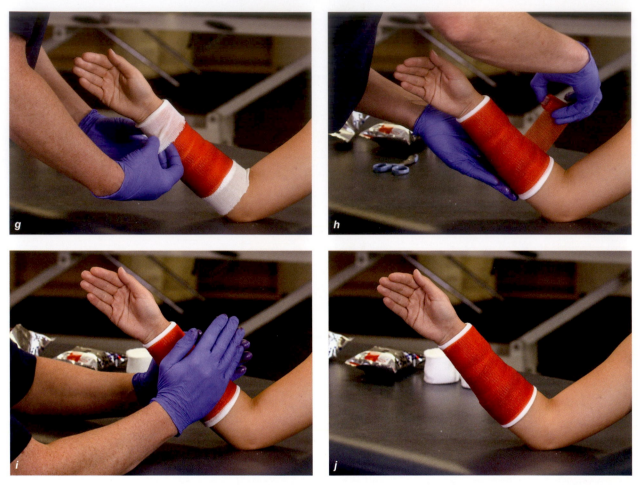

Figure 6.12 *(continued)* *(g)* Fold down the stockinette and *(h)* secure the ends of the stockinette with the final layers of fiberglass. *(i)* Using the palm and heel of your hand, mold the casting material as needed. *(j)* Completed ulnar shaft fracture cast.

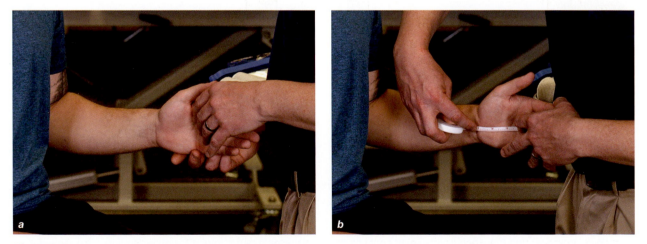

Figure 6.13 Splinting procedure used for a stable forearm fracture. *(a)* Position the elbow in 90º of flexion, the forearm in 0º of pronation, and the wrist in 10º to 15º of extension. *(b)* Measure 4 inches (10 cm) beyond the proximal palmar crease to 4 inches (10 cm) above the antecubital fossa to determine the amount of stockinette needed. *(continued)*

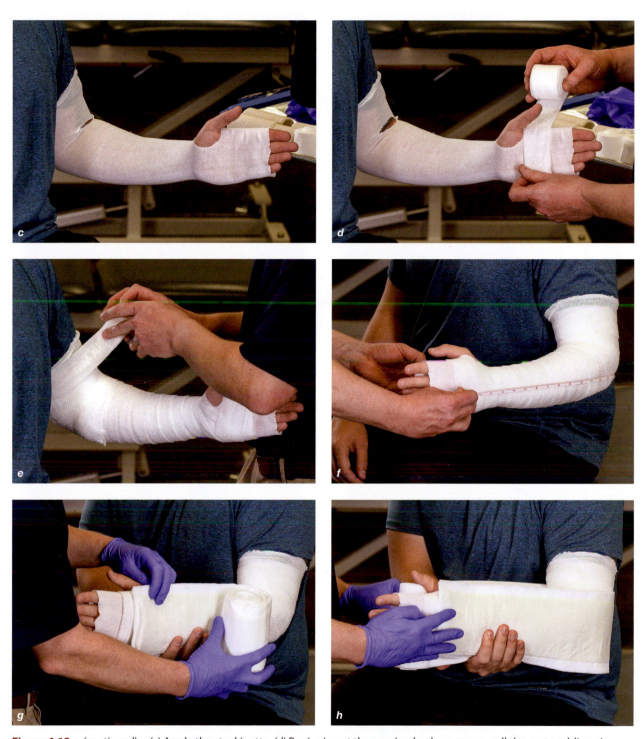

Figure 6.13 *(continued)* *(c)* Apply the stockinette. *(d)* Beginning at the proximal palmar crease, roll the cast padding circumferentially from distal to proximal; *(e)* end by encompassing the elbow in cast padding. *(f)* Starting on the dorsal aspect of the hand, measure from 1 finger width proximal to the MCP joints, around the elbow, to 1 finger width proximal to the palmar crease to determine the length of the splint. *(g)* Starting on the dorsal aspect, position the splint against the hand, wrist, and forearm, *(h)* going around the elbow so the splint contacts the palmar aspect of the forearm, wrist, and hand. *(continued)*

▶ Video 6.6 demonstrates the application of a sugar tong splint for a stable forearm fracture.

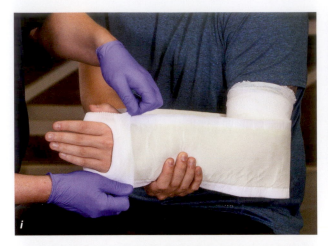

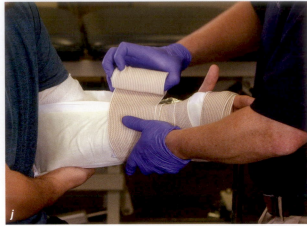

Figure 6.13 *(continued)* *(i)* Fold down any excess splint material. *(j)* Starting distally, secure the splint in place with an elastic wrap. *(k)* Completed forearm sugar tong splint.

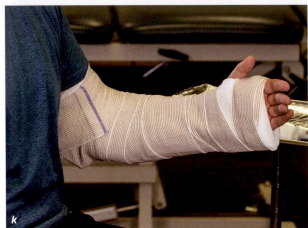

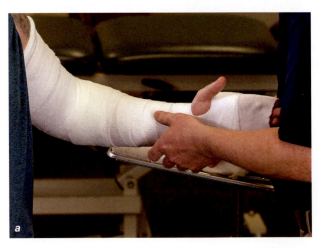

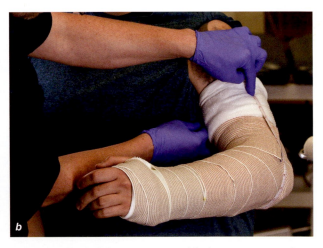

Figure 6.14 Splinting procedure used for an unstable forearm fracture or elbow dislocation. *(a)* Modify the sugar tong splint application by extending the stockinette and cast padding to the base of the axilla. *(b)* Starting at the deltoid insertion, measure around the elbow to 3 inches (8 cm) below the axilla to determine the length of the splint. *(continued)*

 Video 6.7 demonstrates the application of a double sugar tong splint for an unstable forearm fracture or elbow dislocation.

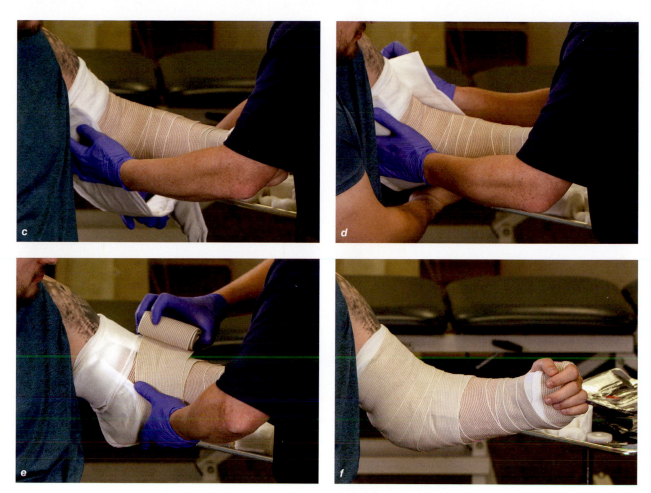

Figure 6.14 *(continued)* *(c)* Begin on the medial aspect by positioning the splint against the upper arm, *(d)* wrapping the splint around the elbow so that it ends at the deltoid insertion. *(e)* Utilizing an elastic bandage, secure the second splint in place by starting below the elbow and moving proximally. *(f)* Completed forearm and elbow double sugar tong splint.

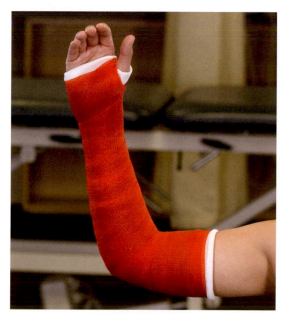

Figure 6.15 Long arm cast.

Video 6.8 demonstrates the application of a long arm cast.

 Visit the web resource for checklists and video clips related to topics discussed in this chapter.

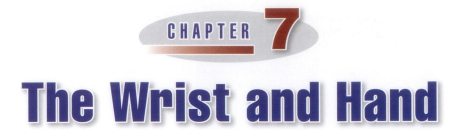

CHAPTER 7

The Wrist and Hand

The wrist has two rows of carpal bones. The proximal row contains the scaphoid, lunate, triquetral, and pisiform bones. The trapezium, trapezoid, capitate, and hamate bones complete the distal row. The hand includes five metacarpal bones, and the fingers have 14 phalanges: a proximal and distal phalanx in the thumb and a proximal, middle, and distal phalanx in each of the four fingers.

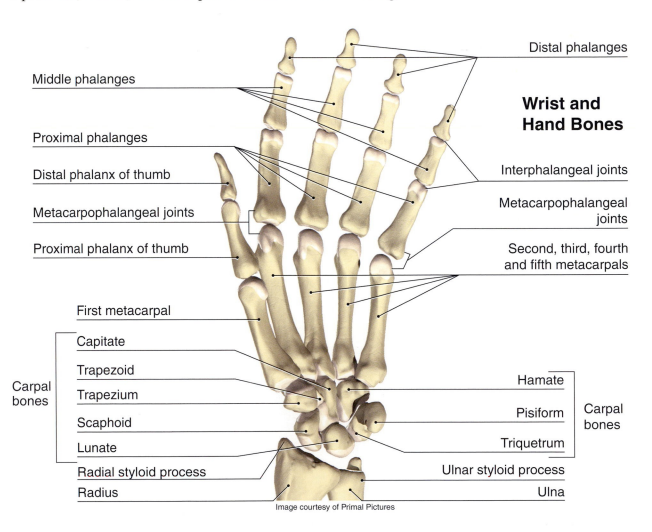

Wrist and Hand Bones

Distal phalanges

Middle phalanges

Proximal phalanges

Distal phalanx of thumb

Metacarpophalangeal joints

Proximal phalanx of thumb

First metacarpal

Interphalangeal joints

Metacarpophalangeal joints

Second, third, fourth and fifth metacarpals

Carpal bones
- Capitate
- Trapezoid
- Trapezium
- Scaphoid
- Lunate
- Radial styloid process
- Radius

Hamate

Pisiform

Triquetrum

Ulnar styloid process

Ulna

Carpal bones

Image courtesy of Primal Pictures

139

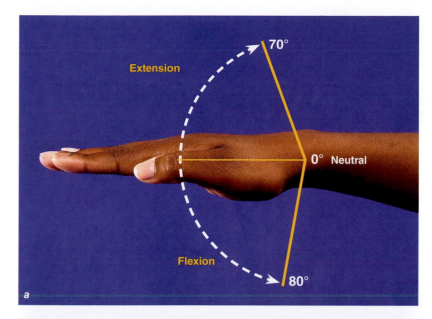

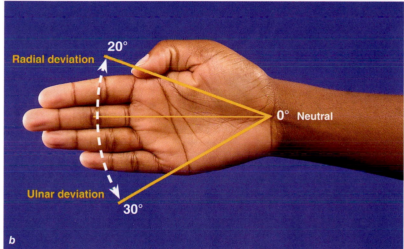

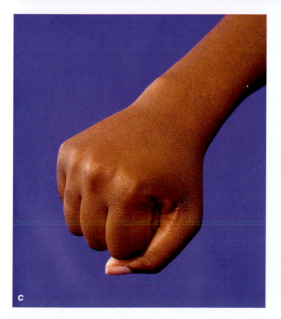
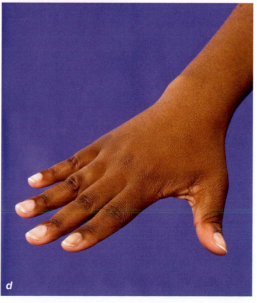

The distal radius and the scaphoid and lunate proximal carpal bones create the wrist joint, allowing movements that include flexion, extension, radial deviation (abduction), and ulnar deviation (adduction) (figure 7.1). The distal carpal bones and the metacarpals form the carpometacarpal joints. The distal ends of the metacarpals and the proximal phalanges of the fingers create the metacarpophalangeal joints. These joints flex, extend, abduct, and adduct. Each of the four fingers contains two joints: the proximal interphalangeal (PIP) and the distal interphalangeal (DIP). The interphalangeal joints permit flexion and extension. A complex network of ligaments and joint capsules supports all the joints in the hand and fingers.

The thumb is crucial because it provides specialized dexterity. The carpometacarpal joint of the thumb permits extension, flexion, abduction, adduction, opposition (figure 7.1), and reposition. The metacarpophalangeal and interphalangeal joints of the thumb permit flexion and extension.

Figure 7.1 *(a)* Wrist flexion and extension ranges of motion; *(b)* wrist radial and ulnar deviation ranges of motion; *(c)* finger flexion, *(d)* extension,   *(continued)*

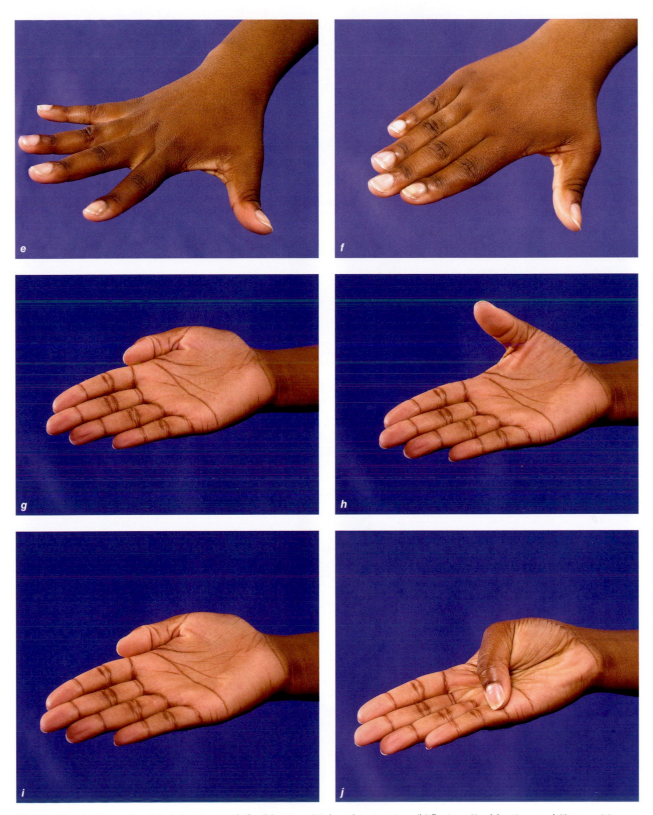

Figure 7.1 *(continued)* *(e)* abduction, and *(f)* adduction; *(g)* thumb extension, *(h)* flexion, *(i)* adduction, and *(j)* opposition.

Ligaments of
the Wrist and Hand

Dorsal carpometacarpal
ligaments

Dorsal intercarpal ligament

Dorsal radiocarpal ligament

Lateral ligament of the
trapeziometacarpal joint

Palmar intercarpal ligaments

Radial collateral ligament

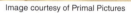

Image courtesy of Primal Pictures

Anterior Forearm

Extensor pollicis brevis

Abductor pollicis longus

Extensor digitorum

Extensor
carpi radialis brevis

Extensor
carpi radialis longus

Pronator quadratus

Flexor pollicis longus

Flexor digitorum superficialis

Flexor carpi radialis

Pronator teres

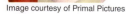

Image courtesy of Primal Pictures

Several ligaments reinforce the joints. The ulnar collateral ligament of the metacarpophalangeal joint, which prevents valgus displacement, needs consideration with respect to athletic injury.

Several muscles originate in the forearm and hand that produce wrist, hand, and finger movement. The flexor carpi ulnaris and the flexor carpi radialis cause wrist flexion, and the contraction of the extensor carpi ulnaris and the extensor carpi radialis longus and brevis produce wrist extension. The simultaneous contraction in the wrist of the flexor carpi ulnaris and the extensor carpi ulnaris results in ulnar deviation. Conversely, if the flexor carpi radialis and the extensor carpi radialis longus contract together, radial deviation occurs. Several muscles that act on the wrist begin from the humerus and cross the elbow joint. They are, therefore, significant for normal function of both the elbow and the forearm.

Three muscles produce movement in the four fingers (figure 7.1). The flexor digitorum profundus and superficialis cause flexion; the extensor digitorum precipitates extension. The flexor digitorum profundus attaches to the distal phalanx of the fingers, and the flexor digitorum superficialis **inserts** into the middle phalanx. The first muscle flexes both the PIP and DIP joints, but the latter muscle flexes only the PIP. Both muscles, however, flex all the joints of the wrist and hand as they pass to the fingers. The insertion of the extensor digitorum gives three tendinous slips to each of the four fingers. A central tendon attaches to the middle phalanx, and two lateral bands pass to the distal phalanx. Along with some of the intrinsic muscles of the hand, this mechanism creates the **extensor hood**.

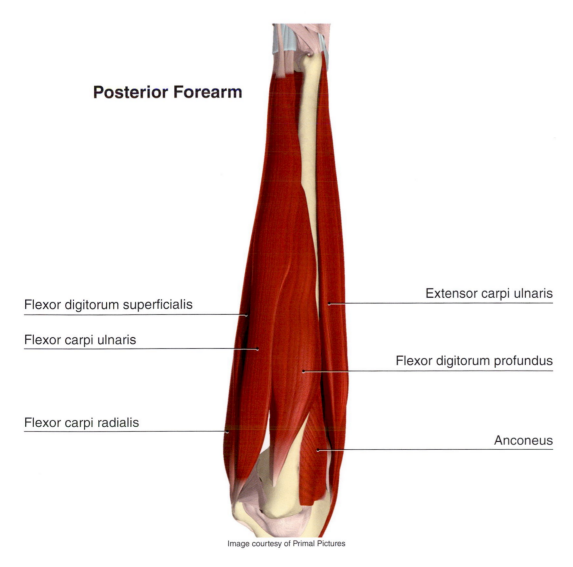

Posterior Forearm

Flexor digitorum superficialis

Flexor carpi ulnaris

Flexor carpi radialis

Extensor carpi ulnaris

Flexor digitorum profundus

Anconeus

Image courtesy of Primal Pictures

Extensor Mechanism of the Finger

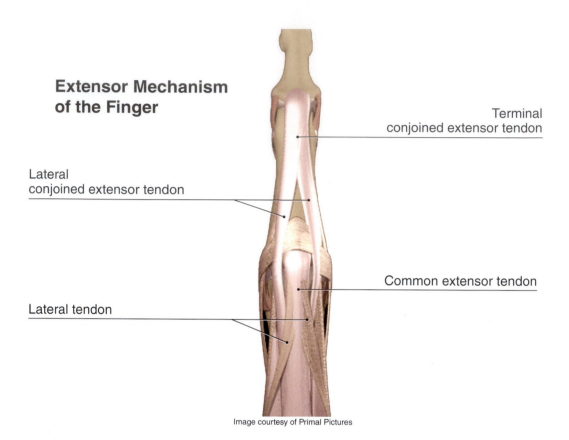

Terminal conjoined extensor tendon

Lateral conjoined extensor tendon

Common extensor tendon

Lateral tendon

Image courtesy of Primal Pictures

Eight muscles act on the thumb to produce its remarkable dexterity. The extensor **pollicis** longus, extensor pollicis brevis, abductor pollicis longus, and flexor pollicis longus originate in the forearm. The extensor pollicis brevis and longus create a space at the base of the thumb, the "**anatomical snuffbox**." The box has clinical significance because the scaphoid bone lies within its borders; point tenderness at this site often indicates a scaphoid fracture. The flexor pollicis brevis, opponens pollicis, abductor pollicis brevis, and adductor pollicis muscles originate in the hand and create the **thenar eminence**, a soft-tissue prominence.

Anatomical Snuffbox

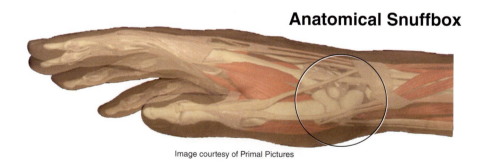

Image courtesy of Primal Pictures

Key Wrist and Hand Palpation Landmarks

Anterior
- ► Pisiform bone
- ► Hook of hamate bone
- ► Thenar eminence
- ► Hypothenar eminence

Posterior
- ► Carpal bones
- ► Carpometacarpal joints
- ► Metacarpophalangeal joints
- ► Interphalangeal joints
- ► Ulnar collateral ligament of thumb

Lateral
- ► Anatomical snuffbox
- ► Scaphoid bone
- ► Radial styloid process

Medial
- ► Ulnar styloid process

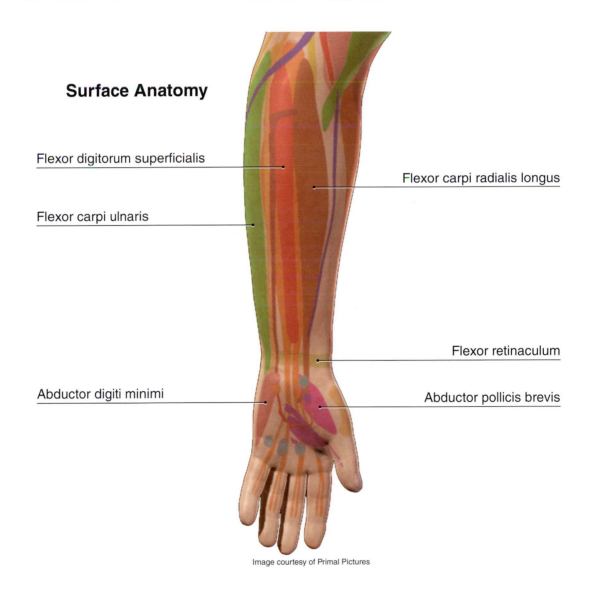

Surface Anatomy

Flexor digitorum superficialis

Flexor carpi ulnaris

Abductor digiti minimi

Flexor carpi radialis longus

Flexor retinaculum

Abductor pollicis brevis

Image courtesy of Primal Pictures

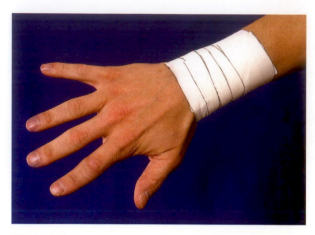

Figure 7.2   Simple wrist taping procedure to limit motion without involving the hand.

WRIST SPRAINS

Wrist sprains often occur when the patient falls on an outstretched hand, causing the wrist either to hyperflex or to hyperextend. Be certain that you have differentiated the wrist sprain from a possible wrist fracture before allowing the patient to return to rigorous physical activity.

Wrist Sprain Taping

Determine whether flexion, extension, or both elicit pain, and apply tape to limit the motion or motions producing discomfort. In some cases, only three or four strips of nonelastic tape around the wrist will be enough (figure 7.2). To prevent a greater range of wrist motion, however, you will have to include the hand in the procedure.

Figure 7.3 illustrates taping that limits both wrist hyperextension and hyperflexion. Place anchors around the wrist and hand and apply a base on the dorsum of the hand using three strips. Follow up by interlocking strips, in an X fashion, over the base. Repeat this procedure on the palmar aspect of the hand. You may then use either elastic or nonelastic tape, applied in a figure-eight pattern around the wrist and hand, to complete the procedure.

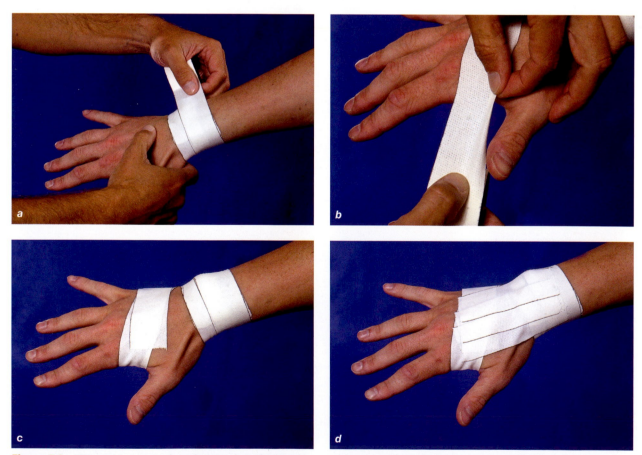

Figure 7.3   Wrist taping procedure that involves the hand to provide greater limitation of motion. *(a-c)* Begin by placing anchor strips around the wrist and hand. *(d-e)* To limit hyperflexion, place three strips and an X over the dorsum of the hand.   *(continued)*

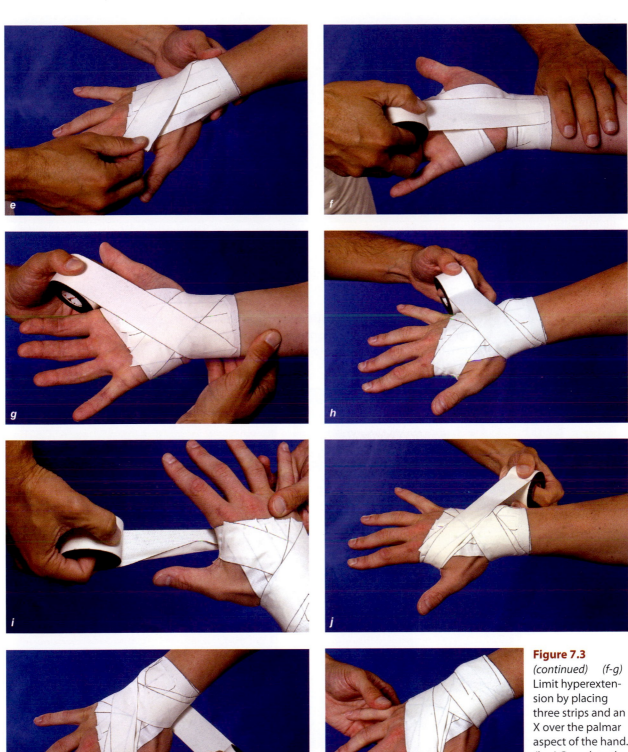

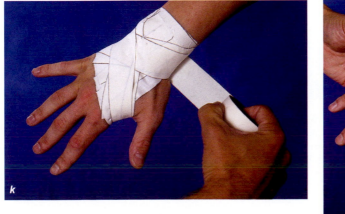

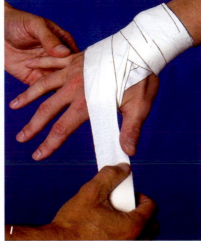

Figure 7.3
(continued) *(f-g)* Limit hyperextension by placing three strips and an X over the palmar aspect of the hand. *(h-n)* Complete the procedure with two figure eights around the wrist and hand. Note in *i* how the tape is crimped to prevent irritation of the webbing of the thumb. *(continued)*

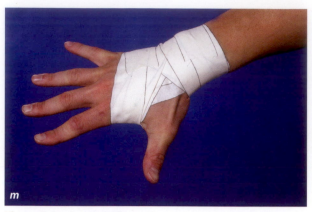
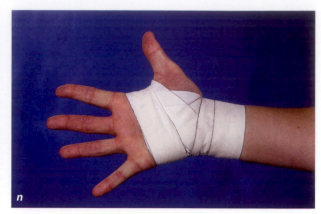

Figure 7.3   *(continued)*

▶ Video 7.1 demonstrates simple wrist and hand taping procedures for hyperflexion or hyperextension sprains.

Strap taping is a more rigid alternative to limiting wrist extension (figure 7.4) or flexion in the presence of wrist sprain or strain. Strap taping can be helpful in limiting pain with epicondylitis related to wrist position.

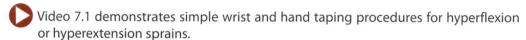

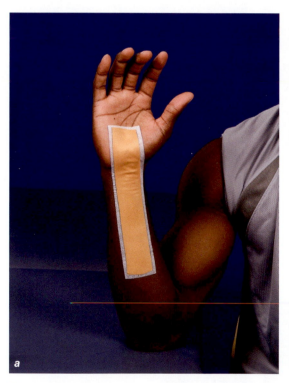
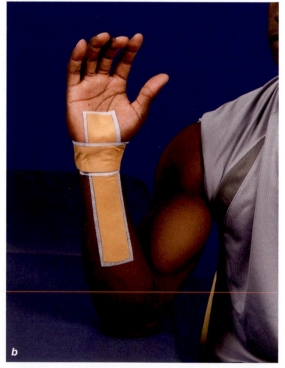

Figure 7.4   Wrist strapping extension block. *(a)* Apply a strip of underwrap with the wrist in neutral position; the strip is applied to the volar midforearm at the level of 1 inch (2.5 cm) distal to the radial styloid process on the palmar hand. Follow with strapping tape, pulling proximally on the volar forearm. *(b)* Apply a second strip of underwrap and strapping tape around the carpals. Ensure the strip around the carpals does not compress the wrist to create or worsen hand paresthesia, pain, or other symptoms.

▶ Video 7.2 demonstrates the strapping tape block technique to limit wrist extension.

Wrist Exercises

Stretch the wrist flexor and extensor muscles with assistance from the contralateral hand (figure 7.5). Hand-held weights will strengthen the flexor and extensor muscles (figure 7.6).

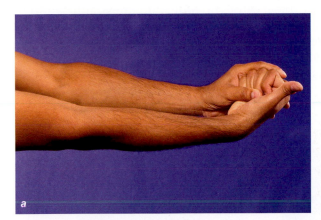
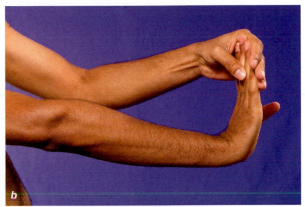

Figure 7.5   Stretching of the wrist *(a)* extensor and *(b)* flexor muscles.

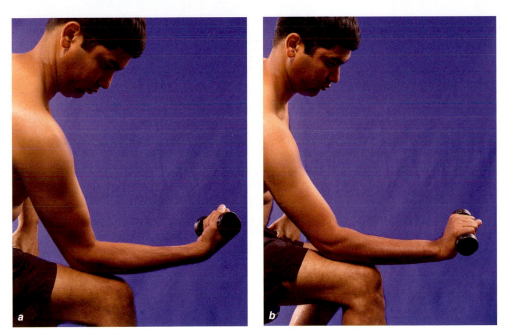

Figure 7.6   Strengthening of the wrist *(a)* flexor and *(b)* extensor muscles with a hand-held weight.

Carpal Tunnel Syndrome

People engaged in activities requiring repetitive motion of the wrist are susceptible to carpal tunnel syndrome (CTS). CTS is compression of the median nerve as it passes through the carpal tunnel of the wrist, and it causes tingling, numbness, and paresthesia in the palm, medial thumb, and first and middle fingers. Musicians, industrial and clerical workers, and even athletic trainers engaged in taping for long hours are susceptible to CTS. A brace designed to protect and rest the wrist from the repetitive stress that produces CTS is commercially available (figure 7.7).

Carpal Tunnel of the Wrist

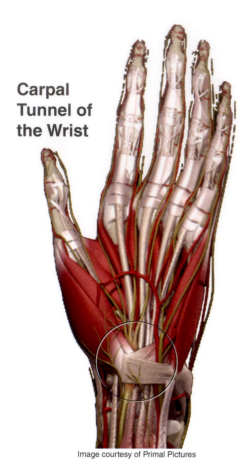

Image courtesy of Primal Pictures

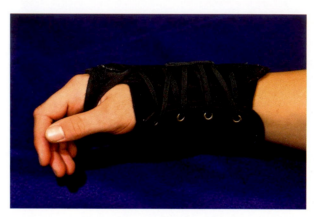

Figure 7.7   A commercially produced brace to relieve the signs and symptoms of carpal tunnel syndrome.

THUMB SPRAINS

Thumb sprains result from hyperextension and involve injury to the ulnar collateral ligament. The colloquial term for this injury is gamekeeper's thumb because the mechanism of ulnar collateral ligament injury was common in gamekeepers who broke the neck of their fowl manually. Injuries that completely rupture the ulnar collateral ligament usually require surgical repair. Partial ligament tears will benefit from a taping procedure.

Rupture of the Ulnar Collateral Ligament of the Thumb

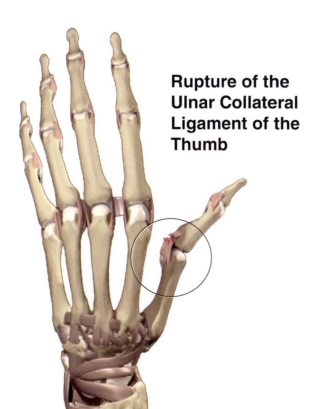

Image courtesy of Primal Pictures

Thumb Sprain Taping

The patient's pain and disability, along with the dexterity that he or she requires, will determine how you proceed. For minor injuries, a simple figure-eight taping around the thumb and wrist will suffice (figure 7.8). If the patient needs the wrist to move freely, begin the individual strips on the anterior surface, encircle the metacarpophalangeal joint of the thumb, and finish on the posterior aspect of the wrist.

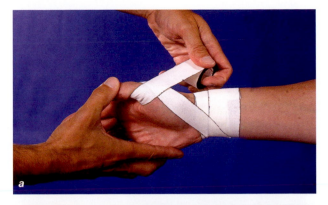

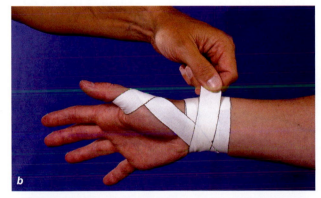

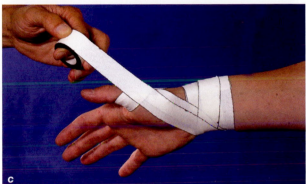

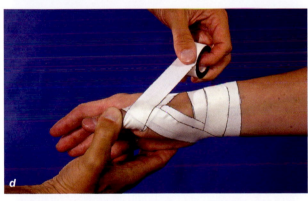

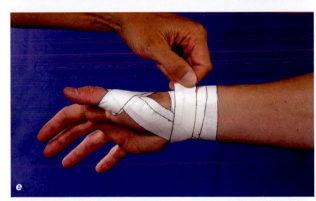

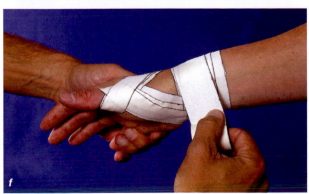

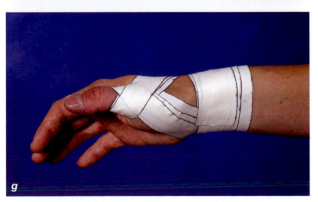

Figure 7.8   Figure-eight taping to support the metacarpophalangeal joint of the thumb. *(a)* Following application of anchor strips around the wrist, begin a strip of tape from the palmar surface of the wrist and proceed around the thumb. Adduct the thumb as the strip passes toward the dorsal surface of the wrist. *(b)* To prevent the bulk that will result from continuous strips around the wrist, individually apply the figure-eight strips. *(c-e)* Successive figure-eight strips overlap the preceding strips in a staircase fashion. *(f-g)* Anchor strips around the wrist complete the procedure.

The procedure for more significant injuries, or for patients who do not need dexterity of the thumb, should incorporate the hand for additional support (figure 7.9). This technique requires anchors at the wrist and hand. Apply figure-eight strips around the thumb and wrist, and overlap horizontal strips from the palmar to dorsal aspect of the hand. These strips will further stabilize the thumb against hyperextension. Complete the procedure with two or three additional figure-eight strips around the thumb and wrist. We do not recommend taping the thumb to the index finger because additional trauma has the potential of injuring the otherwise healthy digit.

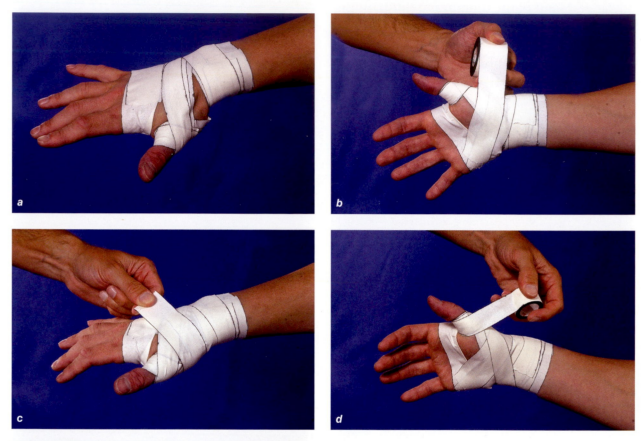

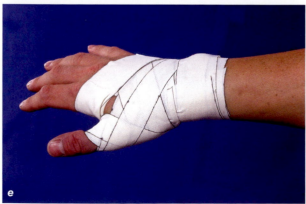

Figure 7.9 Supplement the thumb figure-eight taping procedure with tape that incorporates the hand. *(a)* Following placement of an anchor strip around the hand, *(b-c)* apply strips from the palmar to the dorsal hand anchors over the metacarpophalangeal joint of the thumb. *(d)* Secure these strips with additional figure-eight strips and *(e)* complete the procedure by securing anchor strips around the hand and wrist.

▶ Video 7.3 demonstrates a taping procedure to provide support to a sprained thumb.

Use of an orthoplast spint (figure 7.10*a*) can further stabilize the injured ligament. The orthoplast splint can be positioned (figure 7.10*b*) and secured with elastic tape (figure 7.10*c*).

Kinesiology taping for thumb sprains helps to reduce pain related to extension and abduction movement of the thumb, but does not restrict much motion (figure 7.11). If motion restriction is the goal, use athletic taping instead.

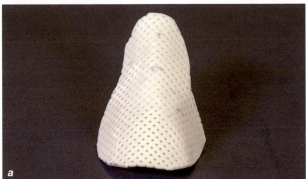

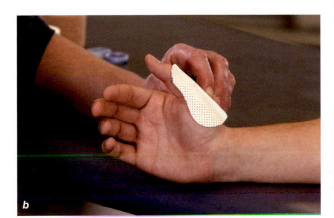

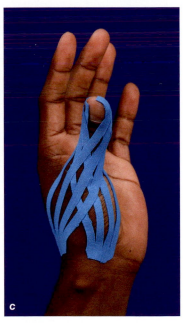

Figure 7.10 *(a)* Cutout of orthoplast splint. *(b)* Placement of orthoplast splint to reinforce thumb taping procedure. *(c)* Orthoplast splint secured with elastic tape.

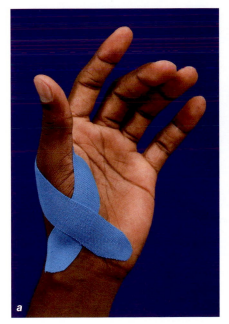

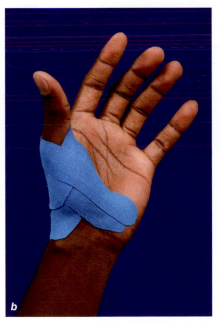

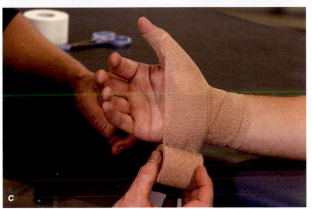

Figure 7.11 Kinesiology taping an ulnar collateral ligament sprain (gamekeeper's thumb). Cut two strips in half lengthwise; each strip should be approximately 6 to 8 inches (15-20 cm) in length. The wrist is neutral and the thumb is in the same plane. *(a)* Start a figure-eight piece at the base of the palmar snuff box, pass through the thumb and index finger web space with tension, and follow along the palmar to ulnar wrist. Tape pieces should overlap at the snuff box. *(b)* Then apply another figure-eight piece around the thumb and wrist with tension but start more distal so the tape crosses distal to the carpometacarpal joint. *(c)* Fan strips are usually the first technique to be applied if swelling is present, and other techniques are layered on top. Use one or two fan strips approximately 4 to 6 inches (10-15 cm) in length to reduce swelling, starting one fan strip proximal to the thenar eminence and fanning toward the metacarpophalangeal (MCP) joint and another fan strip proximal to the first and second metacarpals on the dorsal hand fanning toward the MCP joint.

 Video 7.4 demonstrates kinesiology taping to support a thumb with ligament sprains.

Thumb Exercises

Use the contralateral hand to stretch the muscles acting on the thumb (figure 7.12). Elastic tubing provides an ideal form of resistance for strengthening the thumb and fingers (figure 7.13).

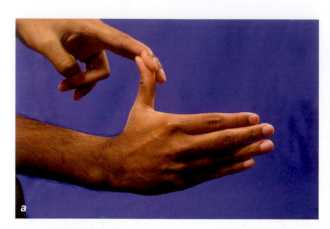 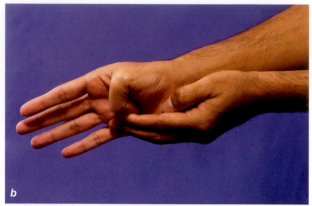

Figure 7.12   Stretching of the thumb *(a)* flexor and *(b)* extensor muscles.

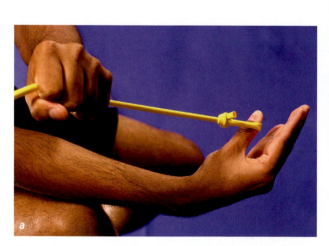 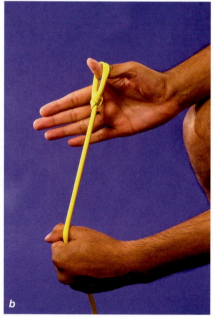

Figure 7.13   Strengthening exercises for the thumb *(a)* flexor and *(b)* extensor muscles with elastic tubing.

FINGER SPRAINS

The proximal and distal interphalangeal joints sprain quite frequently, and their dislocation is the most common form of dislocation injury among athletes. Carefully evaluate finger sprains to make certain that you do not misjudge the injury simply as a jammed finger. Mismanaged fractures, ligament tears, and tendon avulsions will cause significant hand dysfunction.

Finger Sprain Taping

Support unstable fingers by "buddy taping" them to a healthy, adjacent finger (figure 7.14). Tape around the shafts of the proximal and middle phalanges to permit movement at the DIP and PIP joints. If the patient requires gloves, use a collateral ligament taping procedure similar to that illustrated for the knee (see chapter 3). Apply proximal and distal anchors for this technique and continue with interlocking strips, in an X pattern, over the injured ligament (figure 7.15). You will need to tear 1-inch (2.5-cm) tape into smaller widths for this procedure.

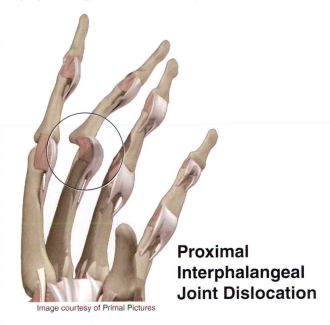

Proximal Interphalangeal Joint Dislocation

Image courtesy of Primal Pictures

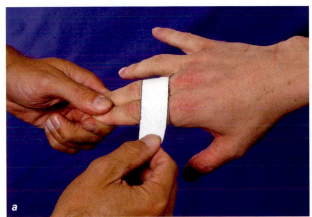

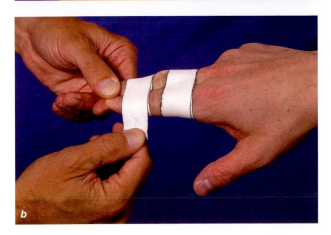

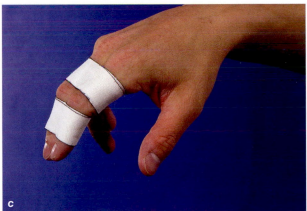

Figure 7.14 Finger "buddy taping." Support the injured finger by taping it to the adjacent finger. *(a-b)* Apply strips on the proximal and middle phalanges. *(c)* Note how the proximal interphalangeal (PIP) and distal interphalangeal (DIP) joints are left open to permit some motion of the fingers while providing support.

 Video 7.5 demonstrates "buddy taping" for support of a finger sprain.

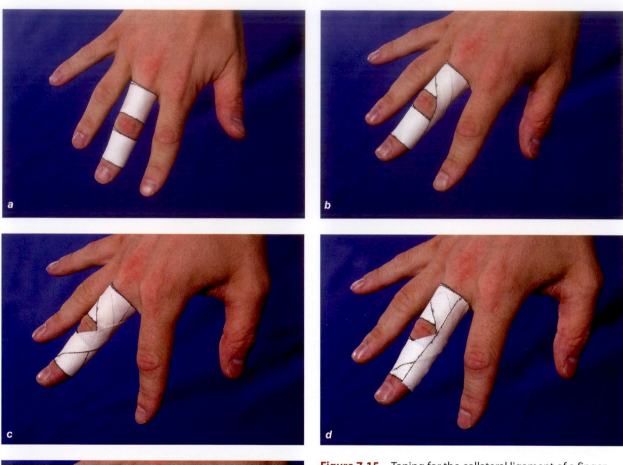

Figure 7.15 Taping for the collateral ligament of a finger. (a) Begin with anchor strips on the proximal and distal finger. (b-d) Create an X over the collateral ligament with three strips of tape. (e) Secure the tape with proximal and distal anchors.

▶ Video 7.6 demonstrates a taping procedure to support the collateral ligaments of the finger.

Finger Exercises

Stretching and strengthening exercises employ the contralateral hand and elastic tubing, respectively (figures 7.16 and 7.17). Squeezing a tennis ball or racquetball will also strengthen the finger flexor muscles.

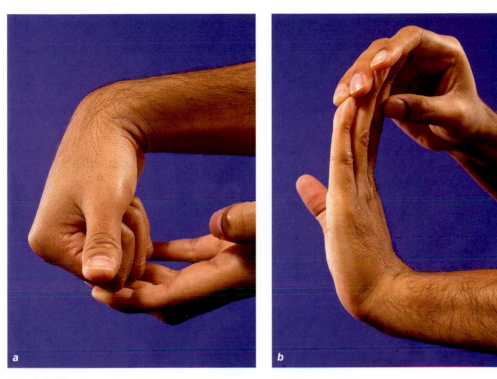

Figure 7.16   Stretching of the finger *(a)* extensor and *(b)* flexor muscles.

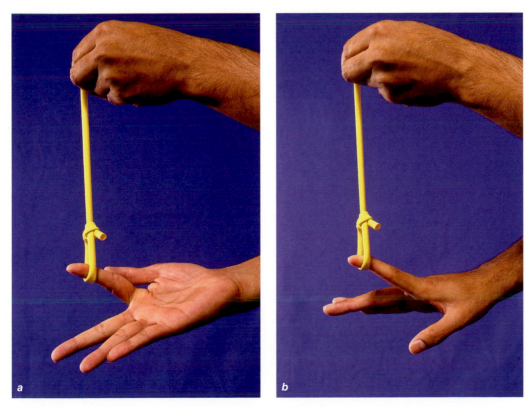

Figure 7.17   Strengthening of the finger *(a)* extensor and *(b)* flexor muscles with elastic tubing.

TENDON RUPTURES AND AVULSIONS

Avulsion of the extensor digitorum tendon from the distal phalanx will force the DIP joint to flex. This injury, colloquially termed **baseball finger**, often occurs when a ball strikes the fingertip.

Tendon Rupture and Avulsion Splinting

Managing the rupture of the extensor digitorum tendon from the distal phalanx involves splinting the DIP in an extended position for 8 to 10 weeks (figure 7.18). Alternate the splint between the palmar and dorsal surfaces of the finger to prevent maceration of the skin. Manually extend the DIP joint while changing the splint, because any joint flexion will require you to restart the immobilization clock.

**Rupture of the Extensor
Digitorum Tendon**

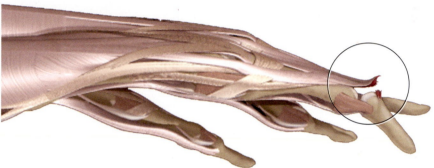

Image courtesy of Primal Pictures

Tendon Rupture and Avulsion Exercises

Have the patient exercise the finger to restore its normal range of motion and strength after the tendon rupture or avulsion heals. Prescribe the exercises illustrated in figures 7.16 and 7.17. An experienced clinician with appropriate medical clearance should both approve the patient to begin the exercises and provide supervision during the regimen.

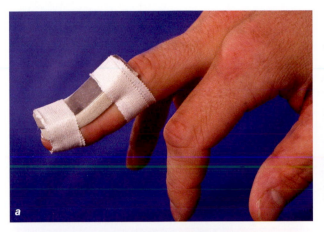

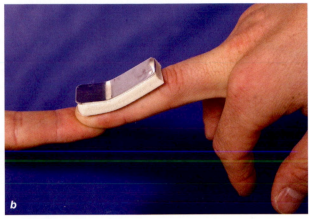

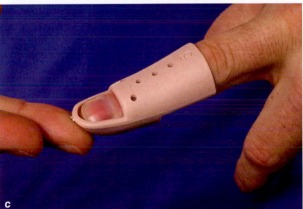

Figure 7.18 *(a)* A mallet finger splint designed to prevent flexion of the distal interphalangeal joint. *(b)* The joint must not flex while you are changing the splint. *(c)* A commercially produced splint can also be used to prevent flexion.

FRACTURES OF THE WRIST AND HAND

Fractures of the wrist and hand include distal radial shaft fractures, scaphoid fractures, and metacarpal fractures. The common mechanism of injury for distal radial shaft fractures and scaphoid fractures is falling on the outstretched hand. Dependent upon the position of the hand, one can either sustain a **Colles' fracture** (wrist hyperextended) or a **Smith's fracture** (wrist hyperflexed). The mechanism of injury for a scaphoid fracture is falling on the outstretched hand with the wrist in the extended position. The clinician can differentiate a distal radial fracture from a scaphoid fracture based upon the area of maximal tenderness. Scaphoid fractures should be suspected and immobilized even if initial radiological findings are negative. Immobilization should be maintained until repeat radiographs are obtained 2 weeks later.

Metacarpal fractures can occur to any of the metacarpal bones, with fracture to the fifth being the most common. Fifth metacarpal fractures are also known as "Boxer's Fractures" because the common mechanism of injury is a force to the metacarpal bone that occurs when hitting an object with a closed fist. Other mechanisms of injury to the metacarpals include direct trauma such as a forceful blow to the dorsum of the hand.

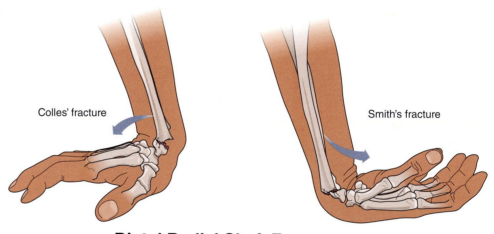

Colles' fracture

Smith's fracture

Distal Radial Shaft Fractures

Scaphoid Fracture

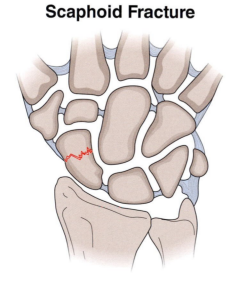

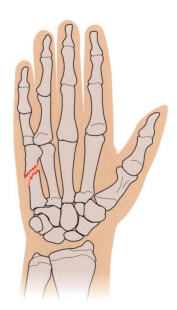

Metacarpal Fracture

Methods for Immobilizing the Fractured Wrist and Hand

Immobilization of the fractured wrist and hand can be accomplished with splints or casts such as an ulnar gutter splint, radial gutter splint, short arm cast, and thumb spica cast. Ulnar gutter splints (figure 7.19) are used to immobilize fractures involving the shaft of the proximal phalanx or the shaft of the middle phalanx of the fourth or fifth digit as well as fractures involving the fourth or fifth metacarpal. Radial gutter splints (figure 7.20) are utilized to immobilize proximal or middle phalangeal shaft fractures involving the second or third digit as well as second or third metacarpal

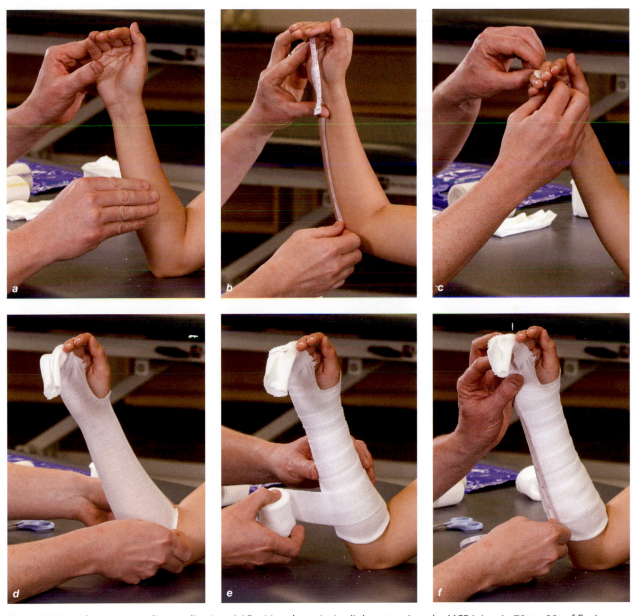

Figure 7.19 Ulnar gutter splint application. *(a)* Position the wrist in slight extension, the MCP joints in 70° to 90° of flexion, and the PIP and DIP joints in 5° to 10° of flexion. *(b)* Measure 2 inches (5 cm) beyond the DIP joint of the ring finger to the antecubital fossa to determine the amount of stockinette needed. *(c)* Place a small piece of cast padding between the fourth and fifth fingers. *(d)* Apply the stockinette. *(e)* Beginning at the DIP joint of the ring finger, roll the cast padding circumferentially from distal to proximal, ending 2 inches (5 cm) below the antecubital fossa. *(f)* Measure from the DIP joint of the ring finger to 2 inches (5 cm) below the antecubital fossa to determine the length of the splint. *(continued)*

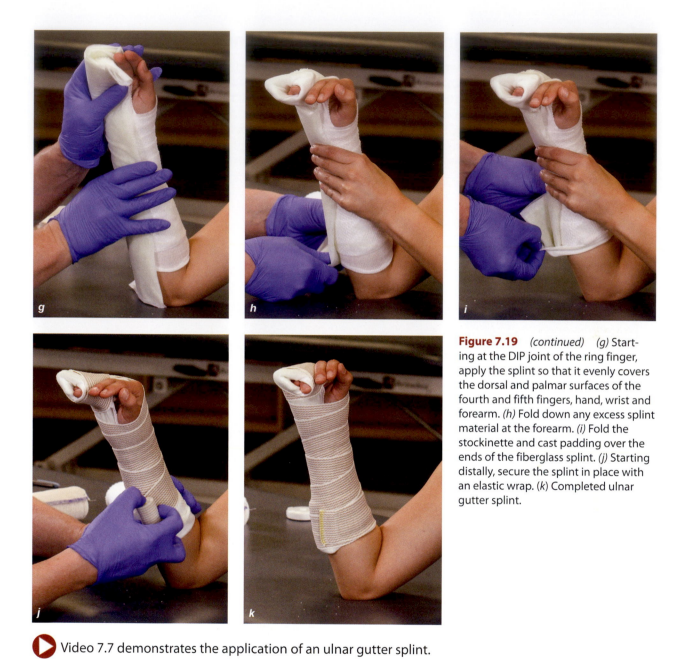

Figure 7.19 *(continued)* *(g)* Starting at the DIP joint of the ring finger, apply the splint so that it evenly covers the dorsal and palmar surfaces of the fourth and fifth fingers, hand, wrist and forearm. *(h)* Fold down any excess splint material at the forearm. *(i)* Fold the stockinette and cast padding over the ends of the fiberglass splint. *(j)* Starting distally, secure the splint in place with an elastic wrap. *(k)* Completed ulnar gutter splint.

▶ Video 7.7 demonstrates the application of an ulnar gutter splint.

fractures. Distal radial fractures are immobilized with a short arm cast (figure 7.21), while fractures involving the thumb, first metacarpal, or scaphoid are immobilized with a thumb spica cast (figure 7.22). A bivalve thumb spica cast (figure 7.23) can be utilized to provide maximum support to soft tissue injuries such as wrist and thumb sprains. The advantage of a bivalve cast is that it can be applied to provide maximal support during practice or competition and removed when not needed.

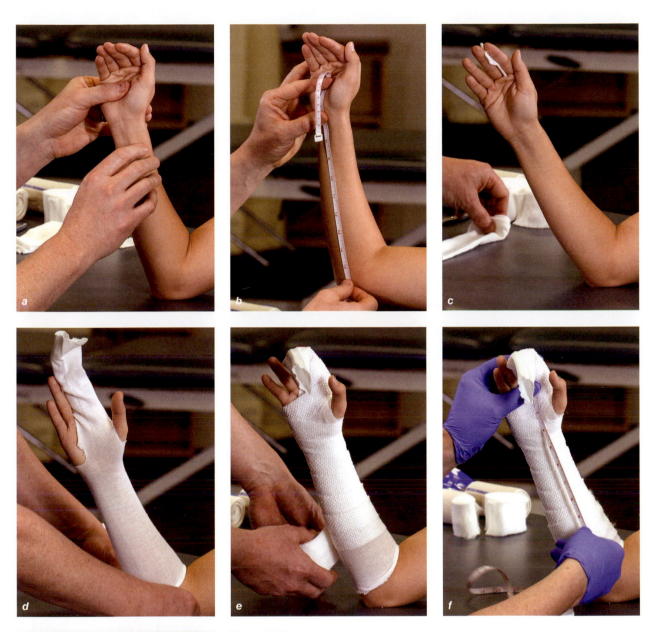

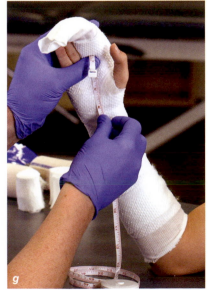

Figure 7.20 Radial gutter splint application. *(a)* Position the wrist in slight extension, the MCP joints in 70° to 90° of flexion, and the PIP and DIP joints in 5° to 10° of flexion. *(b)* Measure 2 inches (5 cm) beyond the DIP joint of the middle finger to the antecubital fossa to determine the amount of stockinette needed. *(c)* Place a small piece of cast padding between the second and third fingers. *(d)* Apply the stockinette. *(e)* Beginning at the DIP joint of the middle finger, roll the cast padding circumferentially from distal to proximal, ending 2 inches (5 cm) below the antecubital fossa. *(f)* Measure from the DIP joint of the middle finger to 2 inches (5 cm) below the antecubital fossa to determine the length of the splint. *(g)* Measure from the DIP joint of the middle finger to the proximal wrist crease and   *(continued)*

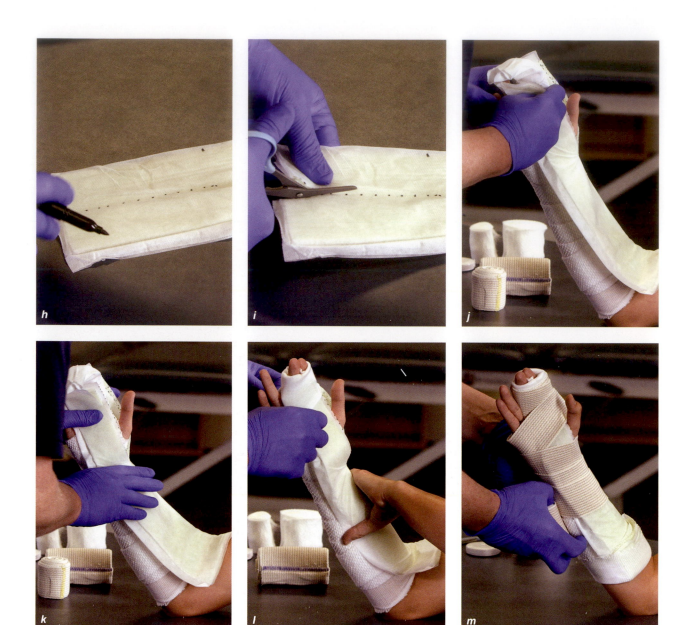

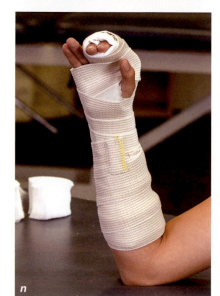

Figure 7.20 *(continued)* *(h)* mark this distance on the splint material. *(i)* Cut down the middle of the splint material to the mark that you just made. *(j)* Starting at the DIP joint of the middle finger, apply the splint with one half on the dorsal aspect of the second and third fingers and the other half on the palmar aspect of the second and third fingers. *(k)* Continue applying the splint, ensuring that the splint evenly covers the dorsal and palmar surfaces of the hand, wrist, and forearm, then fold down any excess splint material at the forearm. *(l)* Fold the stockinette and cast padding over the ends of the fiberglass splint. *(m)* Starting distally, secure the splint in place with an elastic wrap. *(n)* Completed radial gutter splint.

▶ Video 7.8 demonstrates the application of a radial gutter splint.

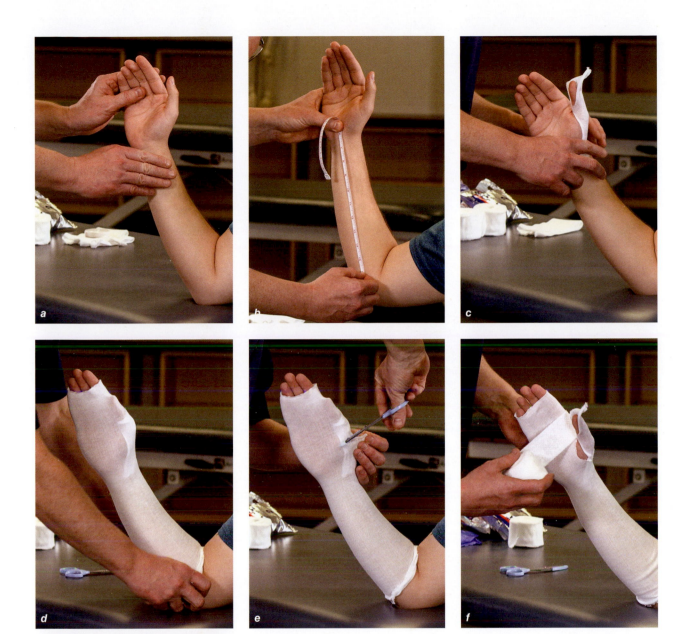

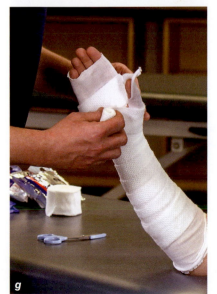

Figure 7.21 Short arm cast application. *(a)* Position the wrist and hand in the "handshake" position with the elbow at 90° of flexion, the forearm in 0° of pronation, wrist slightly extended, and the thumb in neutral. *(b)* Measure from the DIP joint of the middle finger to just above the antecubital fossa to determine the amount of stockinette needed. *(c)* A smaller stockinette is used to cover the thumb. *(d)* Apply the stockinette, and *(e)* cut a small hole in the stockinette over the thumb. *(f)* Beginning at the palmar flexion crease, roll the cast padding circumferentially from distal to proximal, overlapping by 50% to end 3 finger widths below the antecubital fossa. *(g)* Apply extra cast padding around the base of the thumb. *(continued)*

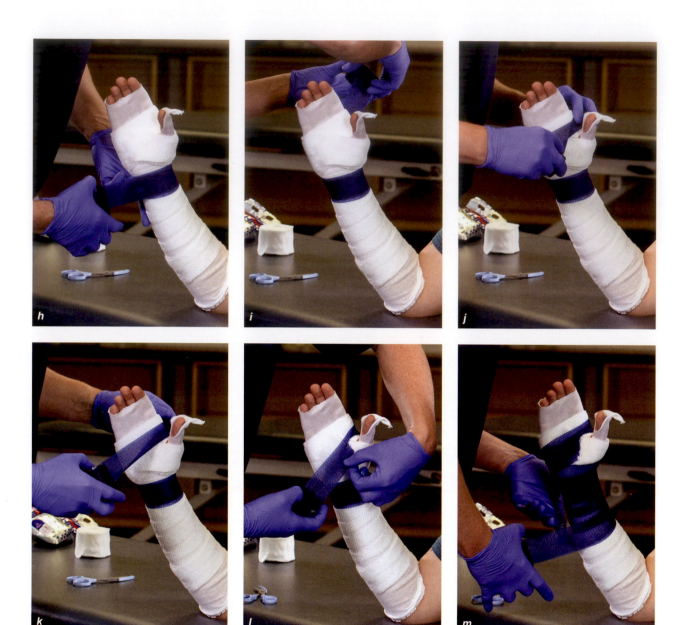

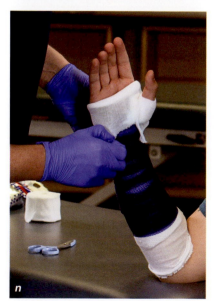

Figure 7.21 *(continued)* *(h)* Start by anchoring the fiberglass at the wrist. *(i)* Transition from the wrist to the hand by wrapping around the ulnar border of the hand. As you wrap the fiberglass over the webspace of the thumb you will need to apply one of three different methods to avoid pinching the thumb: *(j)* twist the fiberglass 180° (1/2 turn), *(k)* pinch the fiberglass, or *(l)* cut a slit in the fiberglass. As you encompass the hand on the dorsal aspect, the fiberglass should not go past the MCP joints. On the palmar aspect, it should not go past the palmar flexion crease. After applying two layers of fiberglass at the hand, *(m)* transition to the forearm and, moving distal to proximal, end the fiberglass in the proximal forearm, making sure each layer overlaps the previous layer by 50%. *(n)* Fold down the stockinette and *(continued)*

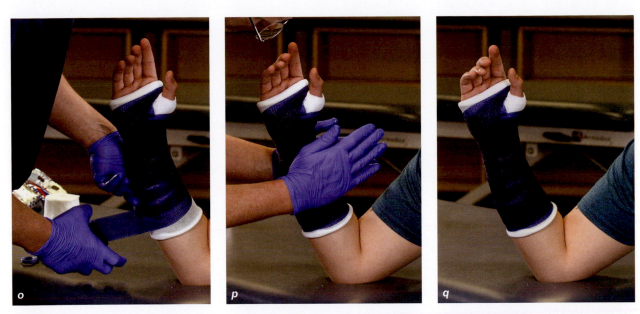

Figure 7.21 *(continued)* *(o)* secure the ends of the stockinette with the final layers of fiberglass. *(p)* Using the palm and heel of your hand, mold the casting material as needed. *(q)* Completed short arm cast.

▶ Video 7.9 demonstrates the application of a short arm cast.

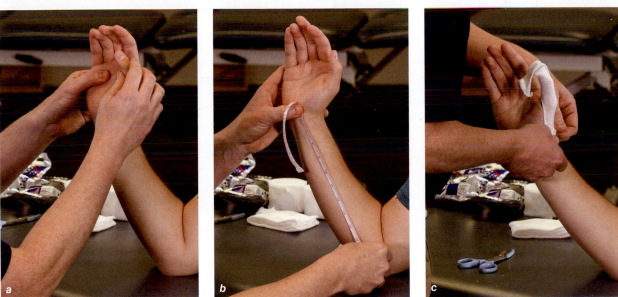

Figure 7.22 Thumb spica cast application. *(a)* Position the elbow in 90° of flexion, the forearm in 0° of pronation, the wrist in 30° of extension, and the thumb as if the patient is "holding a soda can." *(b)* Measure from the DIP joint of the middle finger to just above the antecubital fossa to determine the amount of stockinette needed. *(c)* A smaller stockinette is used to cover the thumb. *(continued)*

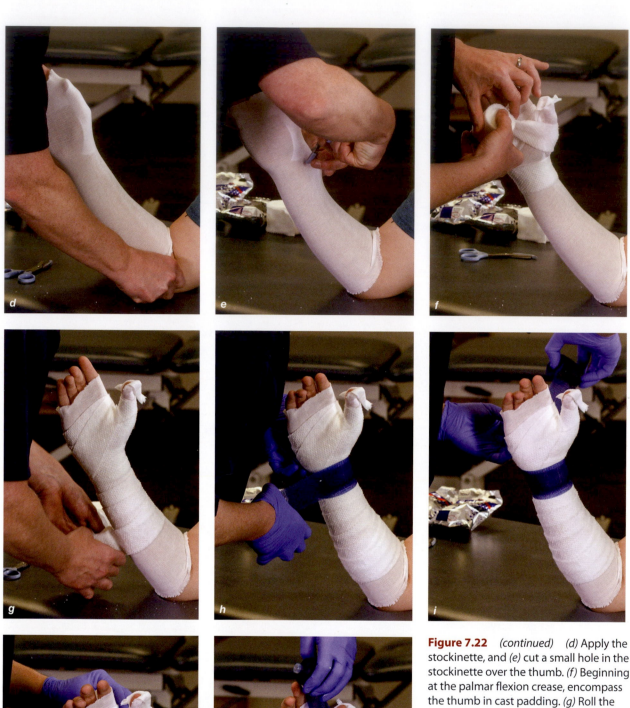

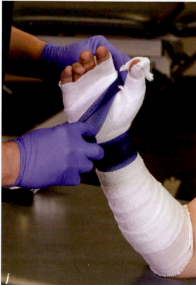

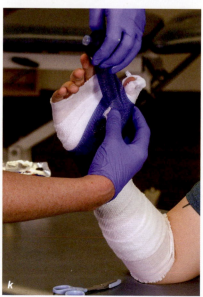

Figure 7.22 *(continued)* *(d)* Apply the stockinette, and *(e)* cut a small hole in the stockinette over the thumb. *(f)* Beginning at the palmar flexion crease, encompass the thumb in cast padding. *(g)* Roll the cast padding circumferentially from distal to proximal, overlapping by 50% to end 3 finger widths below the antecubital fossa. *(h)* Start by anchoring the fiberglass at the wrist. *(i)* Transition from the wrist to the hand by wrapping around the ulnar border of the hand. *(j)* As you wrap the fiberglass over the webspace of the thumb you will need to apply one of three different methods to avoid pinching the thumb (see figure 7.21*j-l*). After completing one layer around the hand, *(k)* transition to the thumb and encompass the thumb with fiberglass. *(continued)*

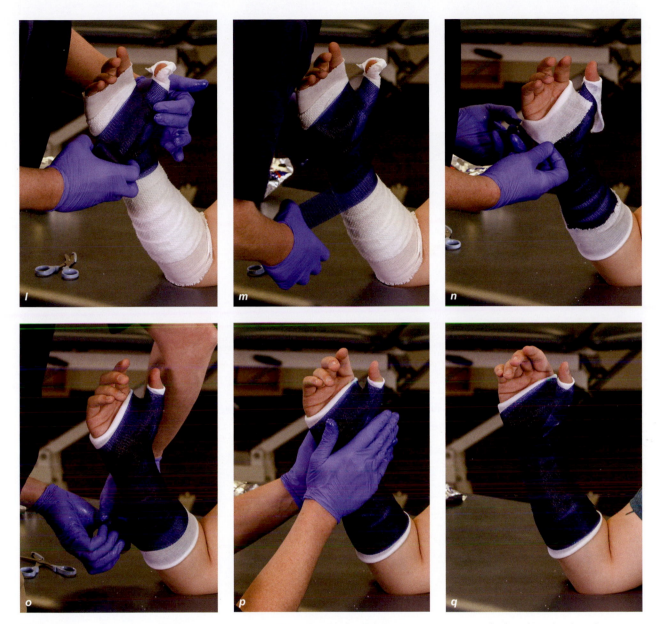

Figure 7.22 *(continued)* *(l)* Apply another layer of fiberglass to the hand. As you encompass the hand on the dorsal aspect, the fiberglass should not go past the MCP joints. On the palmar aspect, it should not go past the palmar flexion crease. After applying the second layer of fiberglass to the hand, *(m)* transition to the forearm and, moving distal to proximal, end the fiberglass in the proximal forearm, making sure each layer overlaps the previous layer by 50%. *(n)* Fold down the stockinette and *(o)* secure the ends of the stockinette with the final layers of fiberglass. *(p)* Using the palm and heel of your hand, mold the casting material as needed. *(q)* Completed thumb spica cast.

 Video 7.10 demonstrates the application of a thumb spica cast.

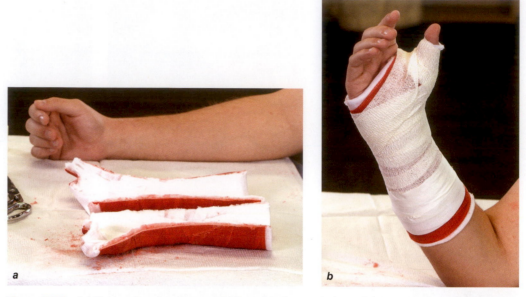

Figure 7.23 *(a)* Bivalve thumb spica cast. *(b)* Securing the two halves of the cast in place with athletic tape.

 Visit the web resource for checklists and video clips related to topics discussed in this chapter.

Glossary

abduction—Movement away from the midline of the body.

acromioclavicular joint sprain—A sprain to the ligaments (acromioclavicular, coraco-clavicular, or both) of the joint formed by the distal clavicle and the acromion process of the scapula; also known colloquially as a separated shoulder.

acute injury—A recent, traumatic injury.

adduction—Movement toward the midline of the body.

anatomical position—Erect position with the arms at the sides and palms of the hands facing forward.

anatomical snuffbox—The space at the base of the thumb created by the extensor pollicis longus and brevis tendons.

antalgic gait—A painful or abnormal walking or running pattern.

anterior—The front or top surface of a limb.

anterior cruciate ligament—A ligament crossing through the knee joint that attaches from the anterior tibia to the posterior femur. The anterior cruciate ligament limits anterior movement of the tibia from the femur as well as rotation of the tibia.

articulation—The point where two or more adjacent bones create a joint.

avascular—The absence of blood supply.

avulsion—The tearing away of a tendon or ligament attachment from bone.

baseball finger—The colloquial term for an avulsion of the extensor digitorum tendon from the distal phalanx of the finger; also known as mallet finger.

biofeedback—Feedback provided through visual observation or an audio tone.

bursa—A fluid sac that reduces friction between two structures.

chronic injury—A nontraumatic injury of an ongoing nature.

circumduction—A combination of abduction, adduction, flexion, and extension.

closed-chain exercise—Exercise in which the distal segment of the extremity is fixed to the ground.

Colles' fracture—A fracture to the distal radius resulting from a fall on the outstretched hand with the wrist in a hyperextended position.

contralateral—Refers to the opposite extremity.

contusion—A bruise.

dislocation—A complete separation of two articulating bones.

distal—A point on an extremity located away from the trunk.

dorsiflexion—Movement of the foot toward the upper, or dorsal, surface.

dorsum—The top of the foot or the back of the hand.

electrical muscle stimulation—Use of electrical current to induce a muscle to contract.

epicondylitis—Inflammation of an epicondyle.

eversion—Outward movement, or turning, of the foot.

exostosis—Abnormal bone growth.

extensor hood—The anatomical tendon configuration on the dorsal aspect of the finger.

extrinsic muscle—A muscle that originates in the leg or forearm and inserts into the foot or hand.

hamstrings—A muscle group in the posterior thigh consisting of the semitendinosus, semimembranosus, and biceps femoris.

hematoma—A collection of pooling blood.

high ankle sprain—An injury involving the anterior tibiofibular ligament and interosseous membrane.

human anatomy—Study of structures and the relationships among structures of the body.

iliac crest—The superior border of the iliac bone; the colloquial term for a contusion to this area is "hip pointer."

innervation—The process of sending a nerve impulse from the central nervous system to the periphery to induce a muscle to contract.

innominate bones—Two flat bones that form the pelvic girdle; each consists of an ilium, a pubis, and an ischium.

insertion—The point where muscle attaches to bone; usually refers to the distal attachment of the muscle.

interdigital—Located between the digits (i.e., the fingers and toes).

intrinsic muscle—A muscle that originates and inserts within the foot or hand.

inversion—Inward movement, or turning, of the foot.

lateral—Toward the outside.

mechanism of injury—Describes the specific cause of the injury.

medial—Toward the inside.

menisci—The intra-articular cartilage of the knee.

myositis ossificans—The formation of bone within a muscle that has suffered a contusion.

open-chain exercise—Exercise in which the distal segment of the extremity does not bear weight.

origin—The point where muscle attaches to bone; usually refers to the proximal attachment of the muscle.

orthotic—A commercially available insert designed to realign and alter the biomechanics of the foot.

overuse injury—Chronic injury resulting from repetitive stress.

periosteum—Outer layer of bone.

pes cavus—A foot with a high longitudinal arch.

pes planus—A foot with a flat longitudinal arch.

plantar fasciitis—Inflammation of the plantar fascia at its attachment to the calcaneus.

plantar flexion—Movement of the foot toward the bottom, or plantar, surface.

plantar neuroma—Inflammation or irritation of a plantar nerve.

pollicis—Pertaining to the thumb.

posterior—The rear or bottom surface of a limb.

posterior cruciate ligament—A ligament crossing through the knee joint that attaches from the posterior tibia to the anterior femur and limits posterior movement of the tibia from the femur.

pronation—Movement of the forearm to place the palm face down; or, while non-weight-bearing, a combination of dorsiflexion, eversion, and foot abduction.

proprioception—Awareness of the position of a body part in space.

proximal—A point on an extremity located near the trunk.

quadriceps (Q) angle—The degree of obliquity of the quadriceps.

quadriceps femoris—The muscle group in the anterior thigh consisting of the rectus femoris, vastus medialis, vastus intermedius, and vastus lateralis.

retinaculum—A soft-tissue fibrous structure designed to stabilize tendons or bones.

rotator cuff—The muscle group in the shoulder consisting of the subscapularis, supraspinatus, infraspinatus, and teres minor.

shin splints—A colloquial term for pain in the leg that can originate from any number of possible sources.

Smith's fracture—A fracture to the distal radius resulting from a fall on the outstretched hand with the wrist in a hyperflexed position.

spica—A figure-eight wrap that incorporates the thigh and hip or the arm and shoulder.

sprain—An overstretching (first degree), partial tearing (second degree), or complete rupture (third degree) of a ligament.

static stretching—Stretching a muscle in a stationary position.

strain—An overstretching (first degree), partial tearing (second degree), or complete rupture (third degree) of any component of the muscle-tendon unit.

subluxation—A partial dislocation of a joint.

superficial—Toward the surface of the body.

supination—Movement of the forearm to place the palm face up; or, while non-weight-bearing, a combination of plantar flexion, inversion, and foot adduction.

surface anatomy—Study of the form and surface of the body.

surgical fixation—The utilization of metal hardware (pins, plates, or screws) to stabilize a fracture.

tendinitis—Inflammation of a tendon or its sheath.

thenar eminence—Intrinsic muscles of the thumb that include the abductor pollicis brevis, flexor pollicis brevis, opponens pollicis, and the adductor pollicis.

valgus—Alignment of a joint or stress to the joint that places the distal bone in a lateral direction; the "knock-kneed" position of the knee joint.

varus—Alignment of a joint or stress to the joint that places the distal bone in a medial direction; the "bow-legged" position of the knee joint.

Bibliography

Abian-Vicen J, Alegre LM, Fernandez-Rodriguez JM, Lara AJ, Meana M, Aguado X. Ankle taping does not impair performance in jump or balance tests. *J Sport Sci Med.* 2008;7:350-356.

Adamczyk A, Kiebzak W, Wilk-Franczuk M, Sliwinski Z. Effectiveness of holistic physiotherapy for low back pain. *Ortopedia, Traumatologia, Rehabilitacja.* 2009;11:562.

Alt W, Lohrer H, Gollhofer A. Functional properties of adhesive ankle taping: Neuromuscular and mechanical effects before and after exercise. *Foot Ankle Int.* 2004;20(4):238-245.

Bragg R, MacMahon J, Overom E, et al. Failure and fatigue characteristics of adhesive athletic tape. *Med Sci Sport Exer.* 2002;33(3):403-410.

Bullard RH, Dawson J, Areson DJ. Taping the "athletic ankle." *J Am Podiatr Assoc.* 1979;69:727-734.

Callaghan MJ. Role of ankle taping and bracing in the athlete. *Br J Sports Med.* 1997;31:102-108.

Capasso G, Maffulli N, Testa V. Ankle taping: Support given by different materials. *Br J Sports Med.* 1989;23(4):239-240.

Cordova M, Scott B, Ingersoll C, LeBlanc M. Effects of ankle support on lower-extremity functional performance: A meta-analysis. *Med Sci Sport Exer.* 2005;37(4):635-641.

Cordova ML, Ingersoll CD, LeBlanc MJ. Influence of ankle support on joint range of motion before and after exercise: A meta-analysis. *J Orthop Sports Phys Ther.* 2000;30(4):170-177.

De La Motte SJ AB, Ross SE, Pidcoe PE. Kinesio tape at the ankle increases hip adduction during dynamic balance in subjects with functional ankle instability. *J Athl Train.* 2009;44:S27-S31.

Delacerda FGPD. Effect of underwrap conditions on the supportive effectiveness of ankle strapping with tape. *J Sports Med Phys Fit.* 1978;18(1):77-81.

Denegar CR, Saliba E, Saliba S. *Therapeutic Modalities for Musculoskeletal Injuries. 3rd ed.* Champaign, IL: Human Kinetics; 2010.

Farrell E, Naber E, Geigle, P. Description of a multifaceted rehabilitation program including overground gait training for a child with cerebral palsy: A case report. *Physiother Theory Pract.* 2010;26(1):56-61.

Feuerbach JW, Grabiner MD, Koh TJ, Weiker GG. Effect of an ankle orthosis and ankle ligament anesthesia on ankle joint proprioception. *Am J Sports Med.* 1994;22:223-229.

Firer P. Effectiveness of taping for the prevention of ankle ligament sprains. *Br J Sports Med.* 1990;24(1):47-50.

Fleet K, Galen S, Moore C. Duration of strength retention of ankle taping during activities of daily living. *Int J Care Inj.* 2009;40:333-336.

Fu T, Wong A, Pei Y, Wu K, Chou S, Lin Y. Effect of kinesio taping on muscle strength in athletes—A pilot study. *J Sci Med Sport.* 2008;11(2):198-201.

Fumich R, Ellison A, Guerin G, Grace P. The measured effect of taping on combined foot and ankle motion before and after exercise. *Am J Sports Med.* 1981;9(3):165-170.

García-Muro F, Rodríguez-Fernández A, Herrero-de-Lucas A. Treatment of myofascial pain in the shoulder with kinesio taping: A case report. *Manual Ther.* 2009;15(3):292-295.

Gehlsen GM, Pearson D, Bahamonde R. Ankle joint strength, total work, and ROM: Comparison between prophylactic devices. *J Athl Train.* 1991;26:62-65.

Genova J, Gross M. Effect of foot orthotics on calcaneal eversion during standing and treadmill walking for subjects with abnormal pronation. *J Orthop Sports Phys Ther.* 2000;30(11):664-675.

González-Iglesias J, Fernández-de-Las-Peñas C, Cleland JA, Huijbregts P, Del Rosario Gutiérrez-Vega M. Short-term effects of cervical kinesio taping on pain and cervical range of motion in patients with acute whiplash injury: A randomized clinical trial. *J Orthop Sports Phys Ther.* 2009;39(7):515-521.

Greene TA, Hillman SK. Comparison of support provided by a semirigid orthosis and adhesive ankle taping before, during, and after exercise. *Am J Sports Med.* 1990;18(5):498-506.

Gross M, Batten A, Lamm A, et al. Comparison of Donjoy ankle ligament protector and subtalar sling ankle taping in restricting foot and ankle motion before and after exercise. *J Orthop Sports Phys Ther.* 1991;19(1):33-41.

Gross MT, Bradshaw MK, Ventry LC, Weller KH. Comparison of support provided by ankle taping and semirigid orthosis. *J Orthop Sports Phys Ther.* 1987;9(1):33-39.

Hadala M, Barrios C. Different strategies for sports injury prevention in an America's Cup yachting crew. *Med Sci Sport Exer.* 2009;41(8):1587-1596.

Halseth T, McChesney JW, DeBeliso M, Vaughn R, Lien J. The effects of kinesio taping on proprioception at the ankle. *J Sport Sci Med.* 2004;3:1-7.

Heit EJ, Lephart SM, Rozzi SL. The effect of ankle bracing and taping on joint position sense in the stable ankle. *J Sport Rehabil.* 1996;5:206-213.

Herrera-Soto JA, Scherb M, Duffy MF, Albright JC. Fractures of the fifth metatarsal in children and adolescents. *J Pediatr Orthop.* 2007;27:427-431.

Hillman, SK. *Core Concepts in Athletic Training and Therapy.* Champaign, IL: Human Kinetics; 2012.

Houglum, PA. *Therapeutic Exercise forMmusculoskeletal Injuries. 3rd ed.* Champaign, IL: Human Kinetics; 2010.

Hsu Y, Chen W, Lin H, Wang W, Shih Y. The effects of taping on scapular kinematics and muscle performance in baseball players with shoulder impingement syndrome. *J Electromyogr Kines.* 2009;19(6):1092-1099.

Hughes LY, Stetts DM. A comparison of ankle taping and a semirigid support. *Phys Sportsmed.* 1983;11(2):99-103.

Jaraczewska E, Long C. Kinesio taping in stroke: Improving functional use of the upper extremity in hemiplegia. *Top Stroke Rehabil.* 2006;13(3):31-42.

Kase K, Hashimoto T, Okane T. *Kinesio Taping Perfect Manual: Amazing Taping Therapy to Eliminate Pain and Muscle Disorders.* Kinesio USA; 1998.

Kase K, Wallis J, Kase T. *Clinical Therapeutic Applications of the Kinesio Taping Method.* Albuquerque NM: Kinesio Taping Assoc.; 2003.

Keetch A. *The effects of adhesive spray and prewrap on taped ankle inversion before and after exercise* [master's thesis]. Provo, UT, Brigham Young University; 1992.

Keil A. *Strap Taping for Sports and Rehabilitation.* Champaign, IL: Human Kinetics; 2012.

Knight KL, Brumels K. *Developing Clinical Proficiency in Athletic Training: A Modular Approach. 4th ed.* Champaign, IL: Human Kinetics; 2010.

Larsen E. Taping the ankle for chronic instability. *Acta Orthop Scand.* 1984;55:551-553.

Lewis JS, Wright C, Green A. Subacromial impingement syndrome: The effect of changing posture on shoulder range of movement. *J Orthop Sports Phys Ther.* 2005;35(2):72-87.

Lohrer H, Alt W, Gollhofer A. Neuromuscular properties and functional aspects of taped ankles. *Am J Sports Med.* 1999;27(69):69-75.

Malina M, Plagenz L, Rarick G. Effect of exercise upon the measurable supporting strength of cloth tape and ankle wraps. *Res Q.* 1963;34(2):158-165.

Manfroy PP, Ashton-Miller JA, Wojtys EM. The effect of exercise, prewrap, and athletic tape on the maximal active and passive ankle resistance to ankle inversion. *Am J Sports Med.* 1997;25(2):158-163.

McGuine TA, Brooks A, Hetzel S. The effect of lace-up ankle braces on injury rates in high school basketball players. *Am J Sports Med.* 2011:39(9):1840-1848.

McGuine TA, Hetzel S, Wilson J, Brooks A. The effect of lace-up ankle braces on injury rates in high school football players. *Am J Sports Med.* 2012:40(1):49-57.

McPoil TG, Cornwall M. The effect of foot orthoses on transverse tibial rotation during walking. *J Am Podiat Med Assn.* 2000;90(1):2-11.

McPoil TG, Cornwall M. Foot and ankle update: Biomechanics, evaluation, and orthotic intervention (course notes, APTA Annual Conference, Denver, CO); 2007.

Meier K, McPoil T, Cornwall M, Lyle T. Use of antipronation taping to determine foot orthoses prescription: A case series. *Res Sports Med.* 2008;16(4):257-271.

Metcalfe RC, Schlabach GA, Looney MA, Renehan EJ. A comparison of moleskin tape, linen tape, and lace-up brace on joint restriction and movement performance. *J Athl Train.* 1997;32(2):136-140.

Mohammadi F. Comparison of 3 preventive methods to reduce the recurrence of ankle inversion sprains in male soccer players. *Am J Sports Med.* 2007;35(6):922-926.

Morris H, Musnicki W. The effect of taping on ankle mobility following moderate exercise. *J Sports Med Phys Fit.* 1983;23(4):422-426.

Murray HL. Effect of kinesio taping on proprioception in the ankle. *J Orthop Sports Phys Ther.* 2001;31:A-37.

Myburgh KH, Vaughan CL, Isaacs SK. The effects of ankle guards and taping on joint motion before, during, and after a squash match. *Am J Sports Med.* 1984;12(6):441-446.

Olmsted LC, Vela LI, Denegar CR, Hertel J. Prophylactic ankle taping and bracing: A numbers-needed-to-treat and cost-benefit analysis. *J Athl Train.* 2004;39(1):95-100.

Paris DL, Vardaxis V, Kokkaliaris J. Ankle ranges of motion during extended activity periods while taped and braced. *J Athl Train.* 1995;30(3):223-228.

Pederson TS, Ricard MD, Merrill G, Schulthies SS, Allsen PE. The effects of spatting and ankle taping on inversion before and after exercise. *J Athl Train.* 1997;32(1):29-33.

Petrisor BA, Ekrol I, Court-Brown C. The epidemiology of metatarsal fractures. *Foot Ankle Int.* 2006;27:172-174

Purcell SB, Schuckman BE, Docherty CL, Schrader J, Poppy W. Differences in ankle range of motion before and after exercise in 2 tape conditions. *Am J Sports Med.* 2009;37(2):383-384.

Rarick GL, Bigley G, Karst R, Malina RM. The measurable support of the ankle joint by conventional methods of taping. *J Surg Bone Joint.* 1962;44:1183-1191.

Ray R, Konin J. *Management Strategies in Athletic Training. 4th ed.* Champaign, IL: Human Kinetics; 2011.

Rezac D, Rezac S. Therapeutic taping theory and application (course notes, APTA Annual Conference, Denver, CO); 2009.

Ricard MD, Sherwood SM, Schulthies SS, Knight KL. Effects of tape and exercise on dynamic ankle inversion. *J Athl Train.* 2000;35(1):31-37.

Robbins S, Waked W, Rappel R. Ankle taping improves proprioception before and after exercise in young men. *Br J Sport Med,* 1995;29:242-247.

Shultz SJ, Houglum PA, Perrin, DH. *Examination of Musculoskeletal Injuries. 4th ed.* Champaign, IL: Human Kinetics; 2015.

Simoneau GG, Degner RM. Changes in ankle joint proprioception resulting from strips of athletic tape applied over the skin. *J Athl Train.* 1997;32:141.

Sitler M, Ryan J, Wheeler B, et al. The efficacy of a semirigid ankle stabilizer to reduce acute ankle injuries in basketball: A randomized clinical study at West Point. *Am J Sports Med.* 1994;22(4):454-461.

Slupik A DM, Bialoszewski D, Zych E. Effect of kinesio taping on bioelectrical activity of vastus medialis muscle. Preliminary report. *Ortop Traumatol Rehabil.* 2007;9(6):644-651.

Stahl A. Fundamentals of kinesiotaping (course notes, APTA Annual Conference, Denver, CO); 2005.

Stiell IG, McKnight RD, Greenberg GH, et al. Implementation of the Ottawa ankle rules. *JAMA.* 1994;271(11):827-832.

Surve I, Schwellnus MP, Noakes T, Lombard C. A fivefold reduction in the incidence of recurrent ankle sprains in soccer players using Sport-Stirrup orthosis. *Am J Sports Med.*1994;22(5):601-606.

Thelen MD, Dauber JA, Stoneman PD. The clinical efficacy of kinesio tape for shoulder pain: A randomized, double-blinded, clinical trial. *J Orthop Sports Phys Ther.* 2008;38(7):389-395.

Vaes PH, Duquet W, Handelberg F, Casteleyn PP, Tiggelen RV, Opdecam P. Influence of ankle strapping, taping, and nine braces: A stress Roentgenologic comparison. *J Sport Rehabil.* 1998;7(3):157.

Vanti C, Natalini L, Romeo A, Tosarelli D, Pillastrini P. Conservative treatment of thoracic outlet syndrome: A review of the literature. *Europa Medicophysica.* 2007;43(1):55-70.

Wilkerson GB. Comparative biomechanical effects of the standard method of ankle taping and a taping method designed to enhance subtalar stability. *Am J Sports Med.* 1991;19(6):588-595.

Wilkerson GB. Biomechanical and neuromuscular effects of ankle taping and bracing. *J Athl Train.* 2002;37(4):436-445.

Yasukawa A, Sisung C. Pilot study: Investigating the effects of kinesio taping in an acute pediatric rehabilitation setting. *Am J Occup Ther.* 2006;60(1):104-110.

Yoshida A, Kahanov L. The effect of kinesio taping on lower trunk range of motions. *Res in Sport Med.* 2007;15:103-112.

About the Authors

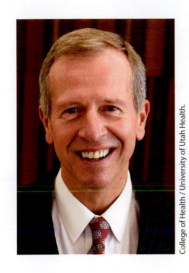

College of Health / University of Utah Health.

David H. Perrin, PhD, FNATA, is dean of the College of Health at the University of Utah and a professor in the department of physical therapy and athletic training. Previously he served as provost and executive vice chancellor and professor of kinesiology at the University of North Carolina at Greensboro (UNCG), after serving as dean of the School of Health and Human Performance at UNCG. Perrin directed the postprofessional master's degree program in athletic training at the University of Virginia from 1986 to 2001. His awards from the National Athletic Trainers' Association (NATA) include the Sayers "Bud" Miller Distinguished Educator Award, the Most Distinguished Athletic Trainer Award, the William G. Clancy Medal of Honor for Research, the Research and Education Foundation's Lifetime Contribution Award, and induction into the NATA Hall of Fame. He is a fellow of the National Athletic Trainers' Association, American College of Sports Medicine, and the National Academy of Kinesiology. For 13 years, Perrin was a member of the NATA Professional Education Committee, helping to write the guidelines for accreditation of both undergraduate and graduate athletic training education programs. He was editor in chief of the *Journal of Athletic Training* from 1996 to 2004 and was the founding editor of the *Journal of Sport Rehabilitation*. He is author of *Isokinetic Exercise and Assessment* and *Athletic Taping and Bracing*, editor of the third edition of *The Injured Athlete*, and coauthor of *Examination of Musculoskeletal Injuries* and *Research Methods in Athletic Training*. In his free time, Perrin enjoys traveling, exercising, and vacationing at his lake cottage in Vermont.

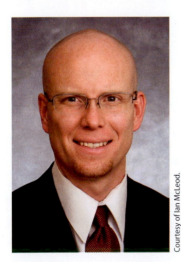

Courtesy of Ian McLeod.

Ian McLeod, PA-C, ATC, is an assistant clinical professor in the department of physician assistant studies at Northern Arizona University. Prior to joining Northern Arizona University, he worked clinically as a physician assistant at University Sports & Family Medicine, part of Dignity Health Medical Group.

Ian's expertise includes athletic training, sports medicine, and primary care. He is a member of the Arizona State Association of Physician Assistants, Arizona State Athletic Trainers' Association, National Athletic Trainers' Association, and American Academy of Physician Assistants. He has extensive experience working with world-class athletes, particularly swimmers. Ian was a member of the U.S. team's medical staff at the 2008 Summer Olympic Games in Beijing. He remains involved with USA Swimming's High Performance Network and has been given the organization's highest honor, the Gold Standard Award. He is the author of *Swimming Anatomy*.

Ian has a master of education degree in athletic training from the University of Virginia as well as a master of science degree in physician assistant studies from A.T. Still University.

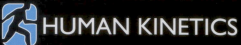
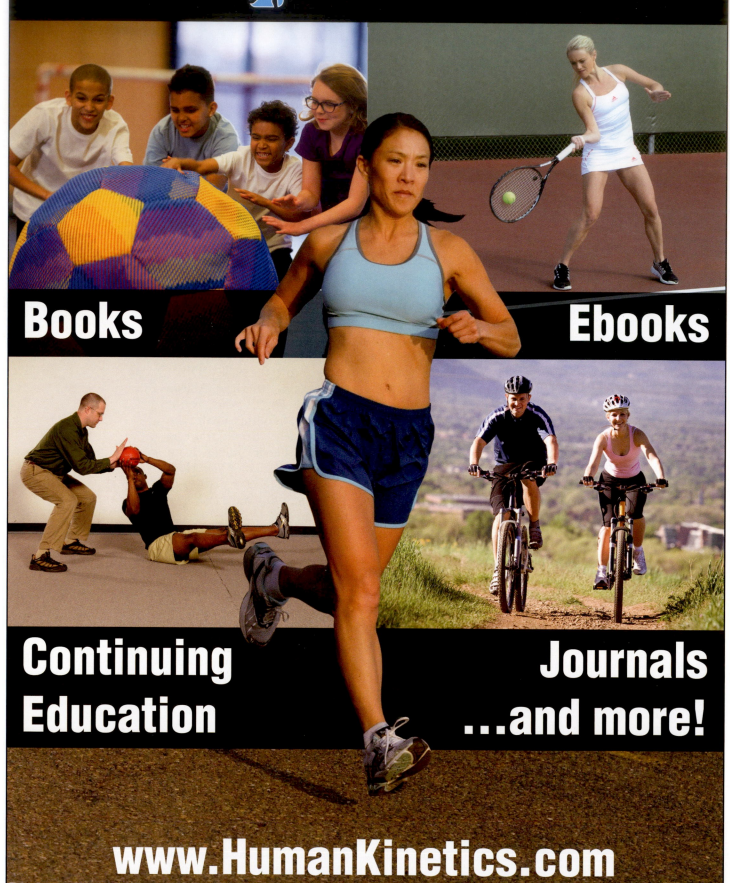

Athletic Taping, Bracing, and Casting

FOURTH EDITION